THE
GOLDEN AGE of
MEDICAL SCIENCE
AND THE
DARK AGE of
HEALTHCARE
DELIVERY

Also by Sylvan Lee Weinberg

An Epitaph for Merlin and Perhaps for Medicine

T H E
GOLDEN AGE OF
MEDICAL SCIENCE
A N D   T H E
DARK AGE OF
HEALTHCARE
DELIVERY

*Reflections on the Practice and
Art of Medicine*

SYLVAN LEE WEINBERG, MD

The Charles Press, Publishers
Philadelphia

The views expressed in this book are not necessarily the views of the American College of Cardiology

The Charles Press, Publishers
Post Office Box 15715
Philadelphia, PA 19103
(215) 545-8933 Telephone
(215) 545-8937 Telefax
mailbox@charlespresspub.com
http://www.charlespresspub.com

Library of Congress Cataloging-in-Publication Data

Weinberg, Sylvan Lee.
The golden age of medical science and the dark age of healthcare
delivery: reflections on the practice and art of medicine / Sylvan Lee
Weinberg.
p. cm.
ISBN 0-914783-90-4 (alk. paper)
1. Medicine — Miscellanea. 2. Medical care — Miscellanea.
3. Medicine — History — Miscellanea. I. Title.
R708 .W3943 2000
610—dc21
00-047436

Printed in the United States of America

First Edition

To all patients whose access to the golden age of medical science has been limited, delayed or denied by the managed care-insurance complex.

ACKNOWLEDGMENTS

To the American College of Cardiology for the opportunity to serve for 15 years as Editor-in-Chief of ACCEL. To William D. Nelligan, Executive Vice President of the College at the time I became Editor-in-Chief, for his confidence and enthusiasm.

To Chris McEntee, current ACC Executive Vice President, for her continued support of the ACCEL enterprise. To Elizabeth Wilson, ACC Assistant Executive Vice President, who was with me from the beginning and who played such a major role in ACCEL's success. To members of the superb ACC Heart House staff who have worked so effectively on ACCEL: Anne Marie Smith; Julie Bainbridge, Managing Editor of ACCEL; Kristen Doermann; and Marcia Jackson, PhD, ACC Associate Executive Vice President for Education. And to Sidney Morton, our longtime Chief Sound Engineer.

To Sylvia Stevens, who has worked with me for many years and throughout my tenure at ACCEL. She has been involved in every manuscript, from first draft to final form. Her expertise and steadfast attention to every detail have been invaluable.

To Lauren Meltzer, Editor-in-Chief of The Charles Press, who edited this book, for her creativity and diligence in meeting the deadline.

To Richard Lewis, MD, MACC, and Dan Ullyot, MD, MACC, Past Presidents of the College, for their review of dozens of editorials, for their help with the final selection and for their enthusiasm and encouragement to publish this volume. To Larry Bonchek, MD, FACC, for suggesting the title. To our distinguished editorial board members — academicians, clinicians and cardiovascular surgeons from around the world — who have contributed so much to the success of ACCEL.

To my wife, Joan, for her candid critique of each editorial and for her indulgence while I was reading, writing and spending so much time overseas acquiring material for ACCEL.

And finally, to our ACCEL listeners for their encouraging response to these editorials, the real impetus for publishing this book.

My thanks and sincere appreciation,
Sylvan Lee Weinberg

CONTENTS

FOREWORD

An eagerly anticipated moment for ACCEL subscribers each month is Dr. Weinberg's editorial. These scholarly, incisive and beautifully worded commentaries have helped make ACCEL an internationally popular and personal educational vehicle. A wide range of topics is covered, from clinical controversies to state-of-the-art presentations related to the ever-changing contents of each issue. These editorials reflect a global view, derived as they are from books and journals worldwide. In fact, Dr. Weinberg was one of the first American educational leaders to recognize the growing importance of cardiovascular research and practice outside the United States. His editorials are always aimed at the practicing physician, reflecting his many years of practice in cardiovascular medicine.

Perhaps even more enduring are the editorials that deal with the complex issues raised by healthcare system reform, including discussions of ethical dilemmas faced by practicing physicians, the adverse impact of "reform" on the training of physicians, the movement toward evidence-based medicine and the use of clinical practice guidelines. Dr. Weinberg has provided highly useful starting points for cardiovascular clinicians who are trying to understand the rapid and dramatic effects of "reform" on their practice.

Many of these editorials have enlightened, if not amused, listeners by describing social and cultural factors outside of medicine that have had effects, often perverse, on the practice of medicine — for example, the influences of Puritanism, the frontier mentality, post-modernism and the challenges of new genetic knowledge. Dr. Weinberg's avid reading outside the field of medicine is reflected in these thoughtful commentaries.

This book is composed of 52 editorials that represent the full spectrum of Dr. Weinberg's commentaries. These essays provide priceless insight into the issues, problems and triumphs of cardiovascular medicine at the end of the 20th century.

Richard P. Lewis, MD, MACC
Professor of Medicine, Ohio State University
Past President of the American College of Cardiology
Columbus, Ohio

PREFACE

The last fifty years have seen enormous progress in medical science — progress that has led to longer life expectancy and better quality of life for Americans. Nowhere is this success story better illustrated than in the prevention, diagnosis and treatment of cardiovascular disease. The development of pharmaceuticals for the treatment of hypertension, hypercholesterolemia, syphilis, streptococcal pharyngitis and heart failure; the development of echocardiography, coronary angiography, cardiac catheterization and nuclear cardiography; and open heart surgery and intracoronary catheter interventions — these are but a few of the scientific advances that have brought great benefit to patients.

Pari passu, the practice of medicine has been transformed from one of close personal relationships between the patient and doctor to a complex labyrinth of specialists, sub-specialists, consultations, laboratory investigations and therapeutic encounters conducted by an increasing number of medical and paramedical personnel. Medical care has also become so expensive that it is beyond the reach of many and, increasingly, beyond the capacity of any insurance scheme, government or private. In its rejection of the 1994 Clinton Health Plan, the American public turned its back on a big government solution to the dilemma of increasingly unaffordable healthcare and instead, it looked to a private sector solution — health insurance coverage through health maintenance organizations (HMOs), which have attempted to hold down medical costs by limiting patients' choice of physician and access to specialty care. However, after nearly a decade of experience with managed care, we now know that Americans are increasingly unwilling to accept limitations of choice and access. After an "inflation lull" during which managed care organizations "low-balled" prices and premiums for the purpose of gaining market share, they were ultimately unable to contain rising medical costs.

In this book of essays, Sylvan Weinberg has captured perfectly the ferment induced by the transformation of cardiologic practice by scientific and technological innovation and the influences of the forces seeking to make medical care affordable. He ranges widely across the panorama of medicine and cardiology, focusing sometimes on exaggerated or misleading inferences about these discoveries, sometimes re-minding us of giants in cardiology, sometimes pointing out how far we have come in a short time, but always leading us with wit and passion to a better understanding of the world we inhabit. Dr. Weinberg is a master essayist bringing historical perspective, a love of language, personal experience in the vineyards of cardiology and an abiding ethical sensitivity to the subjects and issues he addresses in this collection.

It is no exaggeration to say that Dr. Weinberg has acquired a cult following because of his ACCEL editorials, selections from which comprise this valuable, informative and highly entertaining volume. For those who wish to understand current medical science, the limitations of scientific methodology and presentation and, especially, the assaults on professionalism and on the ethical basis of medical practice (the covenant between doctor and patient), I invite you to read this book.

Daniel J. Ullyot, MD, MACC
Director of Cardiovascular Surgery, Mills–Peninsula Hospitals
Clinical Professor of Surgery, University of California, San Francisco
Past President of the American College of Cardiology
Burlingame, California

INTRODUCTION

For the past 15 years, I have had the privilege of serving as Editor-in-Chief of ACCEL, the American College of Cardiology's monthly audio journal. ACCEL (American College of Cardiology Extended Learning) is an international journal of cardiovascular medicine and surgery. Now in its 32nd year, ACCEL was the brainchild of Bill Martz, President of the College in 1969. The first editor was Dale Groom, succeeded in a short time by E. Grey Dimond, President of the College in 1961 and one of the founders of Heart House. Dr. Dimond was editor of the journal for about a decade, during which time he established ACCEL's national presence in American cardiology. He was followed by Bill Likoff, 1967 College President, who was editor until 1985.

Prior to 1990, material for ACCEL was acquired by editorial board members who interviewed leading cardiologists at the annual meetings of the American College of Cardiology and the American Heart Association. At that time, ACCEL consisted of a one-hour tape. Over the past decade, ACCEL has gradually extended its onsite coverage to include the British, French and European Cardiac Societies, and on occasion, the Cardiac Society of Australia/New Zealand and the InterAmerican and Asian-Pacific Cardiac Societies. The editorial board became international and each month's journal tape was increased to three hours. In addition to clinical, research and academic topics, ACCEL also began to explore other issues affecting the practice of cardiovascular medicine and surgery. For example, ACCEL now covers the philosophic, ethical and socio-economic areas that are having a pivotal impact, not only on the practice of cardiology and patient access to care, but also on the funding for research, teaching and support of medical schools and university teaching hospitals.

Over the past several decades, and especially during the past 20 years, scientific progress in cardiology has been spectacular, as it has been in all fields of medicine. In the 1960s, the coronary care unit (CCU) brought a dramatic change to the treatment of patients with acute heart attacks and, in a sense, it introduced the modern era of cardiology practice. But looking back at the CCU, which treated patients with cardiac arrest due to ventricular fibrillation with lidocaine, pacemakers and external defibrillators — important advances at that time — those treatments pale in comparison to what we can do today. Diagnostic catheterization, catheter-based revascularization, bypass surgery, antithrombins, thrombolytics and a myriad of medications have saved and extended the lives of many thousands of patients. Computed tomography, magnetic resonance imaging and echocardiography have further revolutionized our diagnostic approaches. Moreover, the management of atherothrombosis, high blood pressure, stroke and peripheral vascular disease is improving with geometric speed. And now we are at the dawn of a new era in medicine in which molecular biology and genetic-based diagnosis and treatment will make obsolete what today seems so advanced and sophisticated.

But paralleling what can only be called a golden age of medical science, there is what I must reluctantly refer to as a dark age of healthcare delivery. The cost and complexity of our new medical science has put diagnosis and treatment far beyond the financial reach of most people and even, it seems, beyond the reach of government and private sectors. Since the Clinton healthcare debacle in 1994, American healthcare delivery has been dominated largely by private enterprise. Indeed, the much hoped-for equitable distribution and control of healthcare costs by the managed care-insurance complex has failed. It had some initial successes, but its draconian restriction of access to care and specialists did not work. Now, medical costs are once again on the rise. Even in its failure to control rising healthcare costs, the harsh measures imposed by the managed care-insurance complex on hospitals, doctors, patients and university medical centers have had a depressing and chilling effect on every aspect of healthcare in the United States. The doctor's autonomy in making medical decisions has been abrogated. Doctor-patient relationships have been shattered. Many patients have lost access to the doctors and specialists of their choice. Community hospitals and academic medical centers alike, under intense financial pressure from the managed care-insurance complex, have reduced nursing and ancillary staffs and the length of hospital stays, often to the detriment of patient care. Relationships between doctors and hospitals have become strained and at times even adversarial. Some 44 million Americans are uninsured and millions more are underinsured.

At a time when our capabilities to prevent and alleviate disease are so far beyond what could have been dreamed of only a few years ago, our system of healthcare delivery is broken and some believe even fatally flawed. To the paradox of the golden age of medical science and the dark age of healthcare delivery, there is the added irony that this has occurred during a time of unparalleled national prosperity. Perhaps a sign of the times is the title of a recent *New York Times* article: "What If There is No Cure for Healthcare's Ills?"

It is in this milieu — during the rise of medical science and the fall of our healthcare delivery systems — that I have written the editorials collected in this book. I have tried to express the passion of these times — passion for our successes in medical science and passion to find a healthcare delivery system that can bring these successes to all Americans with dignity and without destroying the integrity of the medical profession, our hospitals and our medical schools.

It has been said that much of America's economic success is the result of its distribution system that brings the goods and services of our industry to the people. Thus far, America has not found a similarly successful distribution system for healthcare. Before this can occur there will have to be a sea change in the way medical care is financed. Under the present employer-centered system, the financial intermediary (the managed care-insurance complex) in large measure controls patient access to doctors and hospitals. It also controls vitally important medical decisions. Even in its failure, the managed care-insurance complex extracts far too much money from what is spent on medical care in the United States. This in turn puts financial pressure on hospitals, academic medical centers, doctors and patients, and contributes to what has become de facto medical rationing.

The golden age of medical science is here — still early in its evolution, its potential far from realized — and I remain optimistic that through American ingenuity and sense of fair play, the dark age of healthcare delivery will soon be on the wane.

Sylvan Lee Weinberg, MD, MACC, FESC
Dayton, Ohio
November 2000

Forbidden Knowledge and the Cloning of a Lamb

March 1997

On February 27, 1997, the British scientific journal, *Nature*, published a landmark article of momentous importance, not only to science and medicine, but to all humankind. Entitled, "Viable Offspring Derived from Fetal and Adult Mammalian Cells," the paper is written by Ian Wilmut and his colleagues from the Roslin Institute in Edinburgh. This group was the first to succeed in using the DNA from an adult mammal, a sheep, to create a lamb that was a clone of that adult sheep.

A year earlier, also in *Nature*, the Roslin group reported that they had cloned a sheep by nuclear transfer from a cultured cell line, but in that experiment, embryo-derived cells were used as the nuclear donors. In the current experiment, the genetic material came from a mammary cell of a six-year-old adult sheep. In his article, Wilmut said that the fact that a lamb was derived from an adult cell confirms that differentiation of that cell did not involve the irreversible modification of genetic material required for development to term. The cells in the tissue culture were manipulated so that the DNA became quiescent. The genetic material was removed from an egg cell of another ewe and this cell was in turn fused with a donor cell from the udder of an adult lamb containing all of its DNA. The process involved using a small electrical shock that is perhaps reminiscent of the electricity used by Dr. Frankenstein to give life to his subject in Mary Shelley's classic 19th-century science fiction novel. The developing embryo was then installed in a surrogate mother.

Its potential for good and evil has caused Wilmut's experiment to be compared to the release of nuclear energy. Its possibilities beggar the imagination. Genetic engineering and cloning may create pharmacological proteins with far-reaching potential for treating hitherto untreatable diseases from hemophilia to cystic fibrosis. And there are other prospects not yet even imagined, for example, developing animals with organs that are compatible with human immune systems. This research raises the specter of human cloning with ideas that, until now, were confined to the fertile imagination of writers such as Aldous Huxley and to movies such as *The Boys from Brazil* and Woody Allen's *Sleeper*, which, respectively, involved cloning multiples of Hitler and cloning a world leader from a tissue remnant.

While ethicists and religious leaders ponder the implications of Wilmut's biological breakthrough and while President Clinton bans the use of federal money for cloning humans and related research and calls for a voluntary moratorium by those working with private funds (and predictably, appoints a blue ribbon committee to report within 90 days to tell him what to do), it occurs to me that perhaps the most fundamental issue raised by Wilmut's success is whether or not he and his co-workers have entered that shadowy realm of forbidden knowledge.

One of the most extensive and searching studies of the issues and dilemmas epitomized by Wilmut's classic experiment is a book called, *Forbidden Knowledge: From Prometheus to Pornography*. It was written in 1996 by Roger Shattuck, a former World War II bomber pilot who became Professor of Modern Languages and Literature at Boston University and is internationally recognized in the field of literary criticism. Had Wilmut's work been completed a year earlier, it would have, without question, commanded attention in Shattuck's book.

The first words of Shattuck's foreword define the purpose of his book. He asks, "Are there things that we should not know? Can anyone or any institution in this culture of unfettered enterprise and growth seriously propose limits on knowledge? Have we lost the capacity to perceive and honor the dimensions of such questions?" Thus, Shattuck begins his exploration of man's insatiable desire to conquer the unknown.

Darwin's 1859 *Origin of Species* unleashed a storm of discussion and protest not unlike that which I'm sure will follow Wilmut's experiment. Yet, while Darwin offered a hypothesis or a theory, Wilmut has done something very real to which society will have to respond with more than just the acceptance or rejection of a theory. I trust that our responses to Wilmut's discovery will not mirror that of the Victorian matron, a bishop's wife, who became famous for a remark she made during the controversy on evolution caused by Darwin's ideas. She said, "Descended from apes? My dear, let us hope that it is not true, but if it is, let us pray that it will not become generally known."

Shattuck traces the history of man's attempts to extend human knowledge into the forbidden or unknowable. He begins with Prometheus, the demigod who stole fire from Zeus to help mankind, citing perhaps the most famous pursuit of forbidden knowledge — that which occurred in the Garden of Eden. Other examples he gives are Dante's search for knowledge that lies beyond human knowing and Ulysses' quest as expressed by Tennyson, "yet all experience is an arch through which gleams that untraveled world, whose margin fades forever and forever when I move." Dr. Faust and Dr. Frankenstein also sought to know and to experience the unknowable. And the gentle Dr. Jekyll became Mr. Hyde in his search for what might be called the unknowable or the forbidden. With these and many other allusions to history and literature, Shattuck defines his thesis that mankind's desire for Tennyson's "untraveled world" and for the unknown and perhaps the unknowable is inexorable and cannot be limited or restrained.

After pursuing this theme through legend and literature, Shattuck moves to contemporary scientific reality. J. Robert Oppenheimer, the theoretical physicist who was a driving force behind the World War II atomic bomb project, ultimately became a troubled philosopher when he contemplated the awesome consequences of his scientific success. In 1947, he said, "In some sort of crude sense, the physicists have known sin." When Oppenheimer saw the mushroom cloud of the first atomic bomb exploded at Alamogordo, New Mexico, he quoted from the Bhagavad-Gita: "Now I'm become death, the destroyer of worlds." But in 1994, Edward Teller, another gifted nuclear scientist who also made monumental contributions to the atomic bomb project, said, "There is no case where ignorance should be preferred to knowledge — especially if the knowledge is terrible."

Shattuck contrasts pure science with applied science and reminds us that the disinterested pursuit of science and truth is an activity that will have profound and unpredictable effects when that knowledge is applied. He goes on to tell us how Galileo, Bacon and Copernicus pushed the limits of inquiry and set science on a path of independence from religious restraint. Nicholas Rescher, in a 1984 book entitled, *The Limits of Science*, said, "There seems to be no knowledge whose possession is morally inappropriate per se — here inappropriateness lies only in the mode of acquisition or in the prospect of misuse."

But in spite of all of Shattuck's erudition and searching analysis of mankind's curiosity and thirst for what is not known, he offers no simple solution to his original question about the boundaries of knowledge. Toward the end of the book, he says, "Science and art have enlarged our way of life, but in extreme cases may now endanger it." History leads us back to the question, Are there things we should not know? Shattuck suggests that religion generally says yes and that philosophy generally says no. Although Shattuck returns to this original question several times, he never fully answers it and at the last, he leaves us with a somewhat mixed message. While recognizing a lingering conflict between religion on the one hand and science and art on the other, Shattuck believes that history counsels that science and art should be maintained under what he calls civilian control, warning that Dr. Faust can too easily become Dr. Frankenstein.

Even though Shattuck may be correct that history offers a cautionary view of the limitless expansion of scientific knowledge, and while ethicists and philosophers may ponder these issues and Presidential commissions may render judgments, a more realistic view of history tells us that knowledge and scientific progress will not be restrained. What can be known will be known. What can be done will be done. Thus, society must strive for the proper application of science and knowledge because human curiosity and ingenuity to unveil the unknown will not be contained.

Wilmut's work in Edinburgh may lead to endless benefits — including the control of disease and the transplantation of organs — and yet that same knowledge and technology can be perverted. An enlightened society is not one that suppresses knowledge, but one that learns how to use it appropriately. But this too is patently simplistic because in all facets of human activity, as in medicine, what is appropriate to some is anathema to others. And so will it be with the cloning of the lamb.

2

Genetic Treatment and Enhancement: Prospects Bring Controversy

June 2000

With the completion of the human genome project now looming on the horizon, dramatic changes in the diagnosis and treatment of a wide spectrum of medical conditions must seem inevitable to all but the most skeptical and pessimistic among us. In the March 26, 1999 issue of *Science*, an article by Jon W. Gordon titled, "Genetic Enhancement in Humans" points out that the dramatic progress in gene transfer technology during the past two decades has introduced the possibility of treatment to enhance phenotypic traits. The idea that genetic modification might be used to enhance capabilities in people who are not really suffering from disease has caused tremendous controversy and debate. The prospect that it might even somehow affect human evolution has created philosophic questions that are not easily resolved.

Gordon notes that the term "genetic enhancement" can have different meanings depending on circumstance. The aspect of the controversy that is causing public and academic concern is not that the genetic modification may be used to help reduce disease, but rather that it might be used to augment certain functions in individuals who are not sick — for example, genetically enhancing people to make them excel in athletics or in musical or intellectual pursuits. Another fear is that genetic changes may be transmitted to future generations. Gordon states that while introduced genes can be deleted from germ cells or early embryos from the treated individual, germ line gene transfer has occurred in several animal species and for this reason, any realistic discussion of genetic enhancement must include the possibility of transmission to an offspring. Gordon points out that there has been failure in some animal genetic enhancement studies, for example, the one in which gene transfer in calves initially showed muscle hypertrophy, but then, because degeneration and wasting occurred, it was necessary to kill the animals. Results such as this emphasize that there are still major unsolved problems

5

in gene transfer for enhancement in animals and surely, the same must be true in postulating such procedures for humans.

While understanding is still lacking in the modification of even simple phenotypes, daunting problems obviously remain in more complex areas such as intelligence. The complexity of manipulating intelligence through gene transfer is illustrated by the fact that a single cerebellar purkinje cell has more synapses than the total number of genes in the human genome, and these tens of millions of purkinje cells are involved only in motor coordination. Gordon also tends to debunk the idea that genetic enhancement might in any way affect human evolution. He believes that even if technology were to evolve in the most successful way currently imaginable, only a minuscule number of people would be involved or influenced.

Gordon's impression is that the use of gene transfer for elective enhancement is presently far beyond acceptable or even plausible medical intervention. If there is an attempt to legally ban genetic enhancement, he believes that such procedures could still be performed by conducting them outside the specific areas of jurisdiction. This may be just as well because history tells us that it's far better to prepare society to cope with scientific advances than it is to restrict scientific research. Even if genetic enhancement never becomes feasible, related research is almost certain to make significant progress in the treatment and prevention of devastating and deadly diseases. Gordon concludes that there is potential in this kind of research to improve our understanding of the most complex and compelling phenomenon ever observed — the life process. We cannot be expected to deny ourselves this knowledge. (These issues are reminiscent of the ideas discussed in Roger Shattuck's book, *Forbidden Knowledge*, discussed earlier in this book.)

In spite of Jon Gordon's concession that the experiences of history inveigh against attempts to restrict basic research, on May 24, 2000, the *New York Times* reported that the Clinton administration would seek authority from Congress to level up to a quarter-million-dollar fine on scientists who violate federal laws against human research and a million-dollar fine on the university that employs them. While these fines are ostensibly for violating established procedures, they may very well have an oppressive effect on research initiatives. The Clinton proposals have already faced criticism both on Capitol Hill and in academia. Senator Bill Frist, a cardiovascular surgeon from Tennessee, called them somewhat premature and Gerald Levy, Dean of the UCLA Medical School, said they were radically inappropriate, capable of causing a great deal of chaos and likely to drive people away from doing important research. The severe and restrictive measures proposed by the Clinton administration are probably in response to the highly publicized fatalities of two patients who were receiving gene therapy at major medical institutions.

At the moment, there is a ferment in society regarding these issues. This is quite apparent in the Summer 2000 issue of *Cambridge Quarterly of Healthcare Ethics*, which devotes most of its content to a special section titled, "Breaking Bioethics in Pursuit of Perfect People: The Ethics of Enhancement." It pursues in depth the issues set forth in Gordon's paper with titles such as, "Grand Dreams of Perfect People," "Gene Therapies and the Pursuit of a Better Human," "The Moral Significance of the Therapy-Enhancement Distinction in Human Genetics," and "Are Genetic Enhancements Really Enhancements?"

Norman Daniels, Professor and Chairman of Philosophy at Tufts (who incidentally served on the ill-fated Clinton Healthcare Task Force), draws a distinction between interventions designed to prevent or cure a disease or disability and interventions that are referred to as enhancement in the absence of disease per se. While he mounts what he calls a limited defense of the distinction between treatment and enhancement, his position is ambiguous in that he does not actually give a firm definition of what is disease and what is disability. Thus, he concludes, there are no definable criteria for deciding which genetic interventions are permissible and which are not.

Apparently, I'm not alone in being unable to unravel the specifics of Professor Daniels' position. In his paper, "Grand Dreams of Perfect People," John Lachs, Professor of Philosophy at Vanderbilt, notes, "On careful reading, it's not clear what exactly Daniels hopes to show." At times, philosophers themselves have difficulty interpreting philosophic dissertations. But Lachs' position is quite clear. He takes a rather negative and at best pessimistic view when he says, "Whether it is hubris or foolish hope, we wish to fix everything in the world. Nearly daily reports of progress in mapping the human genome assure us that before long, we'll be able to identify genes for every desirable or undesirable trait. Then we'll be able to obliterate or at least shut down the bad genes and enhance the operation of the good ones to create human beings who will live long, happy and moral lives." And he continues, "Our ignorance is vast and necessary: vast because we are not likely to learn everything we need to know, and we don't really need to know everything we learn; necessary because we can never uncover the secret loves burning in the hearts of others or understand their private hopes and satisfactions." Lachs' goals appear to be more modest than most when he says, "To aim for a little improvement in our children for some small growth in caring, takes the human condition seriously and stands a chance for success." But he believes that large social programs in reengineering the genome will fail, as he puts it, as has every holy war.

And he concludes: "We can walk and sometimes even run, but flapping arms will never make us fly."

David Resnik, Associate Professor of Medical Humanities at East Carolina University School of Medicine, believes that genetic therapy promotes the goals of medicine while genetic enhancement promotes other goals that he considers morally questionable. While he has some difficulty defining medicine's goals with certainty, he does suggest that they include treatment and prevention of disease, promotion of human health and relief of suffering. He believes that genetic enhancement will always be on the slippery slope as to whether it really fits in medicine's province, but that genetic therapy will ultimately be accepted as a part of modern medicine.

From what may be a clinician's simplistic view and from one who tends toward optimism, I would think that genetic treatment and even genetic enhancement will one day become important to medicine in a way far beyond our present ability to predict or even imagine — much as doctors of 60 or 70 years ago would have had great difficulty envisioning the practical application of MRI, thrombolysis, revascularization and many other therapeutic and diagnostic modalities that we take for granted today.

Finally, and not totally unrelated to this discussion, I see that one of my favorite journals, *Perspectives in Biology and Medicine*, until now published by the University of Chicago Press, has been taken over by the Johns Hopkins University Press. In the introductory editorial in the Winter 2000 edition, editors Richard Landau and Robert Perlman write that in 1957, Dwight Ingle, then Professor of Physiology at the University of Chicago, introduced the journal by quoting the great 19th-century English neurologist, Hughlings Jackson, who said: "We have multitudes of facts, but we require, as they accumulate, organization of them into higher knowledge. We require generalizations and working hypotheses." I don't know exactly when Hughlings Jackson said these words (he died in 1911), but they are as applicable today as they were when he said them. Perhaps they are even more applicable today because "multitudes of facts" really doesn't describe the flood of information that is coming to us from multitudinous sources, not least of which is the Internet. Never have we been more in need of organization of those facts into higher knowledge. I'm reminded of a television commercial from one of those financial houses that purports to be able to turn money into wealth. Perhaps our goal by analogy should be to turn facts and bits and bytes of information into wisdom. This may be an illusive goal, but if the information age in which we live and the genomic age now dawning are going to fulfill their promise, somehow, as Hughlings Jackson said, we will have to find the way to turn information into wisdom, however difficult that may be.

3

On *Time to Heal:* Observations and a Review

December 1999

A t the October 1999 meeting of the Canadian Cardiac Society in Quebec City, the moderator announced that one of the doctors he had invited to be on the panel told him that he liked the subject matter of the conference, but that he would participate only if he could be assured that the word "millennium" would not be used. While I applaud that doctor's point of view, I'm afraid that, at this moment, it's not possible to discuss anything great or small without somehow acknowledging that the flow of time has led us to a kind of watershed, however artificial, not only between centuries but between millennia. Nevertheless — and notwithstanding that the third millennium doesn't really begin until the year 2001 — it does seem a good time to contemplate where we have been and where we are going.

While I won't actually deal with the millennium, I will call your attention to a book that is at once timely, scholarly, candid, and I believe, largely accurate in appraising the present state of medicine and the social, political and scientific currents of the past hundred years. The book, *Time to Heal: American Medical Education from the Turn of the Century to the Era of Managed Care*, was written in 1999 by Kenneth M. Ludmerer, an internist, Professor of Medicine and Professor of History at Washington University in St. Louis. Ludmerer begins with a look at medicine in the United States from the turn of the century to the 1910 Flexner report that was commissioned by the Carnegie Foundation for the Advancement of Teaching. Entitled, "Medical Education in the United States and Canada," Flexner's now-classic report excoriated medical education of the time by exposing the fact that it consisted largely of proprietary medical schools that were little more than diploma mills. His report triggered what is now sometimes referred to as a Flexner revolution that caused the proprietary schools of the 1920s to be largely replaced by university-affiliated medical schools with proper laboratories, full-time faculties and effective administrative structures.

The Flexner revolution reversed the deplorable state of American medical education and practice. Implicit in this revolution was a social contract with society that would provide financial, political and moral support for medical education and research and in return, medical schools would serve society. Their success would be measured by the quality of their academic work which would supply America with capable physicians who were dedicated to professionally determined standards.

The classic triad of medical schools, especially since the Flexner report, has been education, research and patient care. However, as Ludmerer very astutely points out, throughout the century, the relative importance of the components of this triad has varied from time to time. For example, between World Wars I and II, education and research were paramount and patient care was pursued only insofar as it was needed to facilitate teaching. Faculties took pride in this new direction and focused on the needs of students, whose education was expanded during the time to include internships and residencies.

During the 1930s, the United States gradually moved to the forefront of medical research and after World War II, research began to replace teaching as the dominant activity, if not the goal, of most medical faculties. This commitment to research was epitomized by the development and expansion of the National Institutes of Health and by 1965, federal grants and contracts accounted for 60 percent or more of the budgets in research-intensive medical schools. Ludmerer calls the time between the great wars the "education era," from World War II to 1965, the "research era" and after 1965, the "clinical era."

With the growth of private insurance after World War II, medical facilities became more and more engaged in what, in reality, was the private practice of medicine. After 1965, with the introduction of Medicare and Medicaid, faculty practice soared when ward and charity patients became paying patients. Within a decade and a half, clinical enterprise eclipsed academic enterprise in most medical schools and faculties generated 50 percent or more of their income from patient care. During each of these three eras — in turn dominated by teaching, research and direct patient care — medical schools expanded tremendously. In 1910, a leading medical school budget may have been around $100,000; by 1940, it was approximately $1 million; by 1965, $20 million; and by 1990, $200 million or more. In the 1980s, medical schools were no longer cohesive organizations and their tripartite mission of education, research and patient care could no longer be held in balance.

Ludmerer makes a point that I think many of you will agree with — that in academic centers in the 1980s, education of medical students, once the unique activity and central mission of medical schools, had become merely a by-product. The ties between medical schools and universities weakened as involvement in healthcare delivery grew. Ludmerer further takes the position that, although through the 1980s education was not really a high priority in medical schools, the quality of medical education remained high. He contends that throughout the century, medical education depended less on a formal curriculum than it did on motivated students who were provided, as he put it, with unfettered opportunities to learn with laboratories, libraries and an ample and diverse supply of patients. And, perhaps most important of all, students had enough time with patients to study them and understand them. But in the late 1980s and 1990s, with the spread of managed care and its growing power and influence, the medical school environment began to change radically and rapidly. Problems with managed care mounted as Health Maintenance Organizations (HMOs) insisted on paying the lowest possible price for medical care. Medical schools were unable to compete with community hospitals because of the inherent high cost of education, research, teaching and certain specialized clinical services that were the hallmarks of medical schools. The decreasing revenues imposed by managed care began to threaten the very viability of the academic centers.

Academic medical centers responded in a variety of ways, but in general, they were forced to expand their clinical enterprise to make up with volume what was lacking in individual patient reimbursement. In effect, more patients had to be seen, meaning that less time could be spent with each patient. Sadly, as Ludmerer doesn't hesitate to say, medical schools and their teaching hospitals, which once measured their success by the doctors they educated and how much new knowledge they produced, inevitably became focused on institutional profitability and clinical market share and began paying less and less attention to what was happening to education and research.

Ludmerer concludes that, without doubt, the quality of academic work in most schools was beginning to suffer as teachers and investigators had to spend more and more time seeing patients while nearly abandoning their educational responsibilities. Further, the quick in and out of patients was wreaking havoc on the learning process and the quintessential feature of medical schools — allowing students and house officers time with patients so as to meet educational needs and objectives — was being lost. In this milieu, a good visit was a short visit. Patients had become consumers and institutional officials looked more at financial sheets than at "relief of suffering." It became an atmosphere that did little to validate the concept of altruism and idealism that students typically bring with them to the study of medicine. In a word, in the late 1990s, what was good for medical schools and faculties was not necessarily good for medical education. Ludmerer also observes that toward the end of the 1990s, faculty practice had many strong advocates among medical school administrators and so, to some extent, did medical research, but education and the teaching of medical students had surprisingly few champions.

Thus, again using that currently unavoidable term, Ludmerer tells us that now, as the millennium approaches, we are in a second revolution in American medicine — one that is characterized by the dismantling of the very infrastructure of medical education that had served so well during most of the 20th century and especially since the first revolution induced by the Flexner report. The educational environment of university medical centers is being eroded and faculty research is decreasing. With regard to the source of faculty salaries, Ludmerer draws a shocking analogy to the proprietary schools of the late 19th and early 20th centuries where faculty income depended mainly on private practice rather than on teaching and research. He contends further that the social contract between society and medicine, and medical school education in particular, has been broken bilaterally, with society no longer providing academic health centers with sufficient financial, political or moral support. In turn, medical faculties have become increasingly unwilling to protect education and similarly reluctant to fulfill traditional responsibilities of standing up for high standards of medical care in the face of managed care constraints.

A further pessimistic observation made in this highly thought-provoking book is that it is really not clear whether medical schools are successfully instilling in students their traditional fiduciary responsibility to patients. To the contrary, in the 1990s, there is growing discussion of how doctors serve the needs of populations, healthcare systems and organizations and surprisingly little is heard from medical faculties about the need for doctors to remain their patients' friend, counselor and advocate.

Ludmerer does concede that, in spite of this, medical schools still rank among the crown jewels of the country's educational system and that the quality of practice still remains high, but the future projections, based on recent trends in medical schools, are very disturbing. The immediate challenge to medical education is somehow to adapt to this rapidly changing marketplace environment without compromising the social contract to provide education and research and to maintain standards of medical care — a goal that, at the moment, is elusive at best.

After a rather dire and foreboding, but I'm afraid accurate, description of what is happening not only to the academic medical center, but also to the entire medical enterprise, Ludmerer literally struggles to end on a somewhat optimistic note by saying that we are still early in the second revolution and there is time, both in and outside the profession, to influence events favorably. He believes that to accomplish this and to restore the social contract between medicine and society, the profession must remember that it exists to serve society and society must remember that it will not have good healthcare unless it provides the needed financial and moral support. Ludmerer suggests that, in the end, society gets the kind of doctors and medical care that it deserves. He believes that while the time left to recapture a constructive initiative is shrinking, there is still sufficient opportunity for visionaries to dream and for leaders to act.

This is a weak ending for a sweeping, powerful and realistic view of American medicine in the 20th century, a century that some have called the health century. Ludmerer's first medical revolution following the Flexner report was a victory for both medicine and society. To the contrary, his second late 20th-century revolution, if successful, will be a defeat for both society and medicine. History tells us that times of great crisis bring forth great leaders with vision and the will to act. World War II produced a Franklin Roosevelt, a Winston Churchill and a Charles DeGaulle. Medicine's second revolution still awaits such leaders. Maybe our crisis is not yet great enough, or perhaps our visionaries are still dreaming and will one day wake up with the will to act.

4

The Uncertainty Principle: From Quantum Mechanics to Medical Education and Practice

January 2000

S everal days ago, while in London after returning from the 10th annual meeting of the French Cardiac Society in Paris, I was fortunate enough to happen upon a riveting and thought-provoking play called "Copenhagen," written by Michael Frayn. The central event in this play is an actual meeting that occurred in Copenhagen in 1941 between two world-renowned theoretical physicists, Neils Bohr and Werner Heisenberg. In the early 1920s, Heisenberg came to Copenhagen to work under Bohr and a close relationship developed between them — Bohr, the distinguished mentor and the younger and brilliant Heisenberg. World War II had put these two great scientists on opposite sides. Heisenberg continued as one of the Third Reich's most eminent scientists working to create an atomic bomb, while Bohr, chafing under the Nazi occupation of Denmark chose to support the Allies for whom he eventually worked at Los Alamos, making significant contributions to the American atomic effort. The central theme of the play swirls around the mystery of why Heisenberg came to Copenhagen in 1941 to meet with Bohr and what happened at that time and in subsequent meetings between the two. The last of these meetings took place in 1947. The play then departs somewhat from history with still another meeting, which although fictional, still leaves many questions unanswered.

I suppose you're probably thinking that none of this has anything to do with medicine, surgery or cardiology, but I think there could be a philosophic analogy between the Heisenberg Uncertainty Principle, which this Nobel Laureate enunciated in 1927, and some issues that are important in the teaching and practice of medicine. Heisenberg's Uncertainty Principle pertains to quantum mechanics and therefore is far beyond my poor power to understand. But simply stated, perhaps too simply, the Uncertainty Principle says that it is impossible to define with precision, simultaneously, the position and momentum of a particle, or to quote Heisenberg directly, "The more precisely the position is determined, the less precisely the momentum is known."

Heisenberg's concept of uncertainty somehow recalls Kenneth Ludmerer's use of the word in his book, *Time to Heal* (discussed in this volume in the editorial entitled, On *Time to Heal*). Ludmerer states that the primary goal of medical education is to prepare students to deal effectively with the uncertainties of everyday practice. He uses the term "training for uncertainty," which he attributes to René Fox, a psychologist who, more than 40 years ago, called this a fundamental aspect of medical education. Ludmerer holds that the most common myth about medical education is that students can learn enough about medicine and disease behavior to be able to act with certainty in every situation. He considers it a fallacy that medical education thinks the uncertainties of the beginner can be replaced with the certainties of the mature physician. Instead, he believes that training students for uncertainty would enable them to practice with intellectual freedom and to be alert for exceptions and then to take a different course of action when warranted by a patient's individual circumstances. Ludmerer quotes a 1932 commission on medical education report that said that a fundamental error in medical education and practice is to consider the human being, who is the unit of medical service, as a uniform standardized organism. Quite to the contrary, no two individuals, even those with the same disorder, react in exactly the same way. Ludmerer decries the lack of training for uncertainty, especially in our current system, which is under severe time restraints imposed by managed care.

It occurs to me that medical education today, perhaps more than ever, assumes that certainty exists and has only to be defined, categorized and promulgated. Ludmerer, on the other hand, believes that uncertainty is inevitable and that a primary goal of medical education should be to train for it. This is the very thesis of Jerome Kassirer, then Editor-in-Chief of the *New England Journal of Medicine*, in a 1989 paper titled, "Our Stubborn Quest for Diagnostic Certainty: A Cause for Excessive Testing." In this editorial, he refers to "our inordinate zeal for certainty." He says, perhaps exaggerating somewhat for emphasis, that "absolute certainty in diagnosis is unattainable no matter how much information we gather, how many observations we make or how many tests we perform. A diagnosis is an hypothesis about the nature of a patient's illness, one that is derived from observations by the use of inference."

Ludmerer describes several principles for educating for uncertainty, including the vital importance of an inquisitive spirit, as enunciated many years ago by George Minot of Harvard, and focusing on individual patients instead of on idealized stereotypes. He further believes that education for uncertainty will ultimately be cost-effective because it will blunt what he calls the misguided quest for certainty that results in diagnostic profligacy. Perhaps even more important is that the concept of uncertainty be recognized as an inevitable part of the medical experience. Not to be aware of the inevitability of uncertainty reduces medicine, in my opinion, to a sterile and anti-intellectual adventure unworthy of any profession.

It is the ubiquity of uncertainty in the human experience that relates medicine to Michael Frayn's play "Copenhagen" and to Heisenberg's Uncertainty Principle, although as I already suggested, it's not possible for most of us to fully understand the milieu in which Heisenberg applied the term. Unresolved uncertainty pervades "Copenhagen." This may be part of its appeal and fascination. There is uncertainty in the wartime relationship and perhaps in the conflict between Bohr and Heisenberg.

Although Heisenberg's Uncertainty Principle is of historic and current significance in the field of quantum mechanics, uncertainty remains, both in the play and in reality, as to whether Heisenberg couldn't or willfully wouldn't consummate the formula that might have given Germany the atomic bomb during World War II. This uncertainty is still being debated today and is pondered in a biography written by David Cassidy entitled, *Uncertainty: The Life and Science of Werner Heisenberg*. In his introduction, Cassidy says that an enormous range of views have been expressed about Heisenberg's activities during World War II and that "for some, the intense emotions unleashed by the unspeakable horrors of that war and [the Nazi] regime have combined with many ambiguities, dualities and compromises in Heisenberg's life and actions to make Heisenberg himself subject to a type of uncertainty principle."

In everyday practice, whether in the operating room, at the bedside, or in our interactions with students and house staff, even as we strive to reduce and limit uncertainty, it may behoove us to remember that Heisenberg's Uncertainty Principle has philosophic significance far beyond the arcane world of quantum mechanics — and not least of all, in our own world of medicine.

5

The American College of Cardiology at 50

December 1998

On December 2, 1949, the American College of Cardiology was granted a corporate charter in Washington, D.C. This last month of 1998 is the first month of a year-long celebration of the 50th anniversary of the founding of the American College of Cardiology.

The unique events surrounding the founding of the American College and its subsequent history are beautifully expressed, both in word and picture, in a 50th-anniversary commemorative volume titled, *The American College of Cardiology: A Visual History, 1949 to 1999.* The 50th-anniversary year officially began on December 12, 1998, at which time this volume was presented at Heart House during a reception and dinner attended by the current and past leadership of the College, including the Board of Trustees, the Board of Governors, the Executive Committee, past Presidents and the College Development and Anniversary Committee, as well as those from industry who have supported the 50th-anniversary celebration in a significant way, and others.

At this event, Richard Lewis, recent past President of the College and Chairman of the 50th-Anniversary Committee, unveiled a magnificent aluminum seal of the College in the Jackie and Simon Dack Atrium at Heart House. Spencer King, current President of the College, presided and introduced Dr. Grey Dimond, President of the College in 1961-62 and one of the founders of Heart House, whose idea it was to create the still state-of-the-art teaching center in the auditorium, where hundreds of cardiologists, nurses and technicians have attended educational programs over the years.

Dr. Dimond, incidentally, was also the first editor-in-chief of ACCEL, prior to the tenure of the late Dr. William Likoff. He recalled vividly and incisively the many obstacles faced by the founders of the American College and the difficulties they had gaining recognition from the leaders of cardiology, many of whom advised their colleagues and fellows not to join this fledgling organization because they saw it as unnecessary and as competitive with the American Heart Association. Fortunately, these conflicts have largely been resolved over the years. These two great organizations now frequently work together, as they did, for example, in the very successful and important drafting of guidelines for the profession. Grey Dimond described a pivotal breakthrough that occurred when he and Paul Dudley White, who once was an opponent of the American College of Cardiology, met by chance in China many years ago. At that time, White encouraged Dimond to bring one of the College's circuit courses to China. Later, Dr. White accepted an honorary fellowship in the College of Cardiology, as did my own revered chief, Dr. Louis Katz, President of the American Heart Association in 1951-52, who had also opposed the College and advised his fellows not to join.

In addition to describing the history of the American College, the 50th-anniversary commemorative volume has an interesting chapter called "The Legacy" that recounts, with broad brush strokes, the evolution of our knowledge of cardiology, dating back to the first comprehensive anatomy text in 1315 from the University of Padua. (Interestingly, more than two centuries later, Andreas Vesalius, also a Paduan professor, drew the depiction of the heart that now appears on the College seal.) There is also reference to René Laennec, James Herrick, Forssmann's cardiac self-catheterization in 1929, and other high moments that have occurred with geometric progression in cardiology over the past 50 years. Mention is also made of other pioneers like Dwight Harken and Charlie Bailey for their work in mitral stenosis; Edler and Hertz for their work in the 1950s that led to clinical echocardiography; and Mason Sones for the first selective coronary angiogram in 1958. And, of course, there is reference to the landmark Framingham Heart Study. Leafing through this volume, one is struck by how many of the procedures that so dominate our cardiology of today occurred during the last 50 years, including: bypass surgery, intracoronary streptokinase, percutaneous transluminal coronary angioplasty (PTCA), the implantable defibrillator, the first coronary stents, radiofrequency ablation, and many other important and classic advances that we now accept so casually. In short, the history of the American College of Cardiology encompasses the history of modern cardiology during the past half century. It doesn't take much imagination to realize that what I've described as geometric progression of cardiology in the past 50 years will seem like slow motion when compared to the progress that will occur during the next 50 years.

It is with this progress in mind that Dick Lewis has orchestrated the "Forum of the Future," to be held in New York City in early in December 1999. At that time, the Board of Trustees of the College will meet — exactly 50 years after the College was founded in that very city. I think it characteristic of the American College of Cardiology that the highlight of the 50th-anniversary celebration will be a look to the future rather than a look to the past. The Forum of the Future, which will be a Bethesda-like conference, will probe the nature and quality of cardiovascular care in the 21st century. Among the issues that it will confront will be the impact of demographics on the change in the practice of cardiology and on physician workforce needs. It will discuss the economics of healthcare and the effective new technology, especially information technology. A consensus summary of the forum will be published in the journal of the American College.

Another part of the 50th-anniversary celebration is the highly successful fundraising campaign which, under the chairmanship of Doug Zipes, has created a fund for the future, generously supported by industry and members of the College, that will be dedicated to educational and communication projects. Further information about the 50th anniversary is published in *Cardiology* (Vol. 27, No. 11, November 1998). During the anniversary year, a series of papers will be reprinted from previous issues of *Cardiology*, along with current commentaries on the significance of medical contributions, how they have stood the test of time, and what changes have occurred. A unique booklet prepared especially for patients will compare treatments and diagnostic techniques in cardiology available 50 years ago with those of today. They should provide a striking contrast.

Perhaps all of us today take for granted the premiere worldwide leadership that the American College of Cardiology has achieved in the field of education and in the care of cardiac patients. We might do well to look back and recall how two immigrant physicians, Franz Groebel and Bruno Kisch, who were already internationally known and distinguished in cardiology, fled Hitler's Germany to resume their careers in New York City. These two cardiologists were later joined by Dr. Phillip Reichert, then a practicing cardiologist in New York City, who became the first Executive Director of the College. In the face of great odds, they were able to establish the American College of Cardiology and guide it through its early years to create the great organization that we know today.

What might be called the modern history of the American College began in 1965 at the annual meeting held in Boston, when Bill Nelligan so impressed Grey Dimond and the late Herman Hellerstein and other leaders of the ACC that he was offered the position of Executive Vice President. But Bill Nelligan, astute and perceptive as he has been throughout his career, made his acceptance contingent upon moving the College from New York City to Washington, D.C. Nelligan's insistence on Washington was accepted and as the saying goes, the rest is history. And part of that history and the history of today is the fact that even at this moment of exhilaration, as we celebrate the first 50 years, cardiology itself and the American College of Cardiology face problems and dilemmas no less daunting than those faced by the founders of the College 50 years ago.

The decade of the 1990s is one of great paradox. While scientific cardiology and our ability to help, heal and even occasionally cure patients is at its zenith, the morale of our profession is at its nadir. This is expressed eloquently in a November 19, 1998 editorial in the *New England Journal of Medicine* by its editor, Jerome Kassirer, titled, "Doctor Discontent." I need not tell you that the despair and discontent to which Kassirer is referring arises from many obstacles that all too often frustrate us in our efforts to deliver our science, skill and even our compassion to our patients. Perhaps the 50th-anniversary challenge to the American College of Cardiology is to achieve the same success that it has had in the education of cardiologists as it confronts the numbing restraints of marketplace medicine on our profession and on our patients. This challenge is no less formidable than the challenges faced by the founders of the College five decades ago. I trust that our success during the next few years will equal theirs of 50 years ago.

6

At the 50th Anniversary of the Irish Cardiac Society: Remembering the Dublin School

October 1999

D r. John Horgan, Chairman of the Program Committee and past President of the Irish Cardiac Society, invited ACCEL to conduct interviews at the 50th Anniversary Meeting and Scientific Sessions of the Irish Cardiac Society in Dublin. Although ACCEL has been privileged to conduct interviews at many national and international meetings around the world, the venue and ambience of the Irish meeting were unique. Instead of studios in the comfortable but rather sterile surroundings of hotel and convention suites, the Irish Cardiac Society interviews were held in the stately and historic home of the Royal College of Physicians of Ireland on Kildare Street in Dublin. This edifice differs little today from the way it looked in the 1860s, shortly after the building was completed.

The building on Kildare Street might never have been, were it not for the efforts of Sir Dominic Corrigan. Corrigan was one of the most prominent physicians of his day and a pivotal figure in what is variously called the "Dublin School" and the "Golden Age of Irish Medicine." The history of this period is admirably described in a book entitled, *Conscience and Conflict: A Biography of Sir Dominic Corrigan, 1802–1880*, written by Dr. Eoin O'Brien in 1983. In his book, O'Brien, a distinguished Irish cardiologist and a devoted and astute student of Irish medical history, describes the Dublin School, which began around 1830, and its remarkable contributions to clinical medicine. According to him, three giants stand out among a galaxy of lesser, though by no means insignificant, luminaries who made up the Dublin School. These men were Robert Graves, Dominic Corrigan and William Stokes. In 19th-century Dublin, there was, as O'Brien put it, a dynamic idealism and iconoclasm that brought a renaissance to Irish medicine and later caused it to gain international recognition.

21

Graves, Corrigan and Stokes had several outstanding talents — a compelling desire to observe the pattern and effect of illness with impartiality (even when their studies refuted conventional practice), the ability to describe their observations with authority and elegance, and the courage to stand up in the face of established medical custom and doctrine. They also traveled abroad frequently and maintained contact with continental and American colleagues. Both Stokes and Corrigan studied in Edinburgh, a leading medical center of the day. One of their teachers and role models was Professor Alison, known equally for his clinical acumen and his dedication to the sick and the destitute, both of which are qualities that characterized the Dublin School. While Corrigan's name is best remembered today for the waterhammer pulse of aortic insufficiency that has come to be known as "Corrigan's pulse," many would be surprised to learn that much of his writings were on scrofula, a name once given to a form of tuberculosis. Corrigan spoke out against the practice of the time of treating already debilitated patients by purging, vomiting, blistering and leeching. Instead, he advocated building the patient up, stopping the vomiting so that strength was not broken down and prescribing "medicaments not rejected," to use his own words. Corrigan's interests went far beyond medicine and later in his career, he served as a Member of Parliament at Westminster.

O'Brien points out that Robert Stokes was the first doctor outside continental Europe to recognize the importance of the stethoscope. He also wrote the first English-language paper on the stethoscope, which René Laennec had first described in 1818. In addition to being an outstanding clinician, Stokes was broadly educated in the arts. Today, he is remembered primarily for two papers he wrote, one of which describes the ominous breathing pattern in patients with advanced cerebrovascular disease. Stokes generously included John Cheyne's name to describe this type of periodic breathing because he recalled that many years earlier, Cheyne had referred to the phenomenon. Both doctors earned a kind of immortality because of Stokes' nearly perfect word picture: "The inspirations become each one less deep than the preceding until they are all but imperceptible and then the state of apparent apnea occurs. This at last is broken by the faintest possible inspiration, then the effect is a little stronger until, so to speak, the paroxysm of breathing is at its height only to subside by a descending scale." This description illustrates the incisiveness of observation and the clarity of expression so characteristic of the Dublin School. While many today may use the term Cheyne-Stokes respirations, few are aware of its origins, but inevitably, such are the limitations of eponymic immortality. In 1846,

Stokes related syncopal attacks to a slow heart rate and again, generously, he gave credit to a prior observation made by Robert Adams, with whom he shares the eponym Stokes-Adams syndrome.

Stokes was ahead of his time, as were other members of the Dublin School, in emphasizing the humanities in the education of medical students and doctors. He said, "Medicine is not a single science — it is an art depending on all sciences." In Stokes' day, there was some opposition to medical specialization. He said of specialization that it would "at best produce a crowd of mediocrities with no chance, or but a little one, for the development of the larger man." Of course, specialization has matured a great deal since Stokes' time, but there is still an element of truth in what he said, perhaps implying mediocrity not related to the specialty, but to the total person.

Robert Graves, the third member of the Dublin School triumvirate, was also a clinician and bedside teacher who had studied in the great centers of Europe before coming back to Dublin. When Graves was in Paris, the great French clinician Trousseau so admired the description Graves gave of hyperthyroid disease in his 1843 book that he proposed that exophthalmic goiter be called Graves' disease. Graves was very sensitive to the interests of his patients. He once warned against the premature discharge of hospitalized patients, saying, "how injurious to persons so debilitated [is] the change from the warmth and comfort of the hospital to the cold and desolation of a damp garret or cellar." Graves added that such practices might improve the hospitals, but at a crucial price. Reading between the lines of Graves' comments, it's difficult to escape the conclusion that even in Victorian Dublin, doctors and patients felt the pressures of cost containment, although I'm sure this phrase was never used. Perhaps they too contended with a managed care-insurance complex, Victorian-style.

Less famous members of the Dublin School were Frances Rynd, who invented the hypodermic syringe which allowed morphine to be given by injection rather than by mouth, and the surgeon, Abraham Colles, who is remembered for the fracture of the wrist that bears his name today. Typical of the Dublin School, Colles was an iconoclast who challenged the Hunterian idea that secondary syphilis was not contagious.

Beginning around 1830, the Dublin School lasted for a mere 50 years. One can only speculate as to what brings about such a flowering of greatness to an institution or to a country, which then, with equal mystery declines, never to be forgotten but perhaps never to occur again. Eoin O'Brien believes that the school was inspired by Graves, Stokes and Corrigan and the coterie of doctors who surrounded them.

He attributes much of the genesis of the Dublin School to the stimulation that these men received through their travels abroad and to the ideas that they brought back from the European capitals of medicine.

O'Brien's book, *Conscience and Conflict*, is well worth reading, not only for its insight into the Dublin School, but also because it is a beautifully written history of 19th-century Ireland, and to some extent England, and of the events and forces that have had such a profound influence on subsequent medical and political history. Of Dublin medicine, O'Brien says, "Had later generations been prepared to seek and absorb the influence of European and American medicine, the school might have survived and Irish medicine might have been saved from a period of stagnation after which it only now shows feeble signs of emerging." While O'Brien's judgment may seem harsh, he is probably correct that moments of greatness are unlikely to occur in a milieu of parochialism and insularity. While we will probably never fully understand what forces conspired to create the Dublin School in the mid-19th century, my observations on the 50th anniversary of the Irish Cardiac Society lead me to believe that, at this time, there is certainly no milieu of parochialism or insularity here. I would not be at all surprised to see a rebirth of the Dublin School in the 21st century.

7

The Quest for Medical Certainty

June 1996

E ven the most casual observer of the polemics in today's cardiology — whether the issue be lipid lowering, the use of stents, angiotensin-converting enzyme (ACE) inhibitors or the superiority of catheter or surgical revascularization — cannot deny that the final arbiter of what constitutes the best practice, not only in cardiology but in all phases of medicine, is likely to be a number or a statistic rather than clinical intuition or judgment. To find support for this thesis, one need only open a medical journal or attend a scientific meeting. The clinical trial is virtually unchallenged as the standard for today's practice.

Most of us probably assume that the clinical trial, as we know it today, dates from the World War II era and Austin Bradford Hill's classic clinical trial to determine the effectiveness of streptomycin for tuberculosis, a study that he designed for the medical research council in Great Britain. While the modern era of clinical trials probably did indeed begin with this study, the struggle leading to the ascendancy of the clinical trial dates back to the early decades of the 19th century and perhaps even before. This process is beautifully and dramatically expressed by J. Rosser Matthews in a book titled, *Quantification and the Quest for Medical Certainty*, published in 1995 by Princeton University Press. Matthews has a doctorate in the history of science from Duke University, and although he is not a physician, he has admirably traced the evolution of medical practice and the development of the clinical trial. I am intrigued by the way he relates the use of numbers — quantification, as he puts it — to the quest for medical certainty, which is really the ultimate goal of clinical research.

In his introduction, Matthews points out that even though the clinical trial has been in the forefront of medical research for only the past generation or two, the use of comparative clinical statistics has had a very long and stormy history. He cites crucial debates that began in the 1830s among clinicians in the Paris Academy of Medicine and continued in 20th-century England, culminating in the first great randomized trial — Bradford Hill's streptomycin for tuberculosis. Matthews' book describes what he calls medicine's Probabilistic Revolution, an effort that continues today as we seek to define probability by new standards of precision and objectivity through the medium of the clinical trial.

The controversy in Paris in the 1830s began between Dr. Pierre Charles Alexander Louis, who sought to use numerical or statistical methods to give the clinician scientific status, and his antagonist, Dr. d'Amador, who maintained that medicine was an art and not a science. Actually, this argument — which perhaps is not yet fully resolved even today — began before the 1830s. It dates back to the later decades of the 18th century, which was the twilight of the Enlightenment, and to the last years of the old regime in France under Louis XVI, who had appointed Marie Antoinette's personal physician to collect statistical data in an effort to stem a cattle plague in 1774. In the 1830s debate, some contended that quantitative reasoning was merely an intellectual distraction to the art of medicine. Dr. Louis, however, was steadfast in invoking the mathematical theory of probability and he was more concerned with collecting empirical facts than with abstract theorizing. It was Louis who in 1853 used a clinical trial to disprove current dogma that bleeding was a cure for pneumonia. Of the 47 patients who were bled, 18 died, while only 9 of the 36 patients who had not been so treated died. Louis' opponent, Dr. d'Amador, challenged the value of statistics, using the example of maritime insurance to illustrate why he thought numbers were not applicable to medicine. He cited this example: If a hundred vessels sink for every thousand that embarked, one would still not know which particular ships would sink. Almost 150 years later, we still have the same problem when we're deciding whether to treat 100 patients to help perhaps 5 or 10, even though we don't know which patients will benefit.

In the 1860s, the great French clinician Trousseau rejected Louis' argument that the doctor should become a kind of empirical scientist. Trousseau believed in the primacy of clinical training and that any type of scientific data must be subordinate to learning how to diagnose and treat the sick. He rejected the numerical method, not because it failed to offer insights into treatment, but because it was used to justify the claim that medicine is a science and not an art. To him, the numerical method implied that there could be exact results, and this notion, he felt, would usurp the power of the intellect. Referring to the numerical method, Trousseau said, "I spurn it with all my energy when it pretends to be a method complete in itself, capable of conducting us to truth." Claude Bernard accepted Louis' vision of medicine as a science, but he saw this science as focused on the individual physiologically deterministic organism. Bernard rejected Louis' numerical method because, among other things, he believed that medicine had to be based on certainty and not on probability. For him, this certainty could come from the experimental laboratory. Also, Louis remained focused on the group rather than on the individual, although he didn't deny, as some of his critics charged, that each patient is individual and unique.

Moving on to England in the early part of the 20th century, Matthews discusses the British Biometrical School and the emergence of Major Greenwood as perhaps the first modern medical statistician. He also describes the intellectual insights of Francis Galton, who studied medicine at Cambridge. Galton's innovations in the statistical method were carried on by Carl Pearson, who went on to teach modern statistical techniques at University College in London. But the going was very difficult for the new breed of biomedical statisticians. In 1901, Galton and Pearson founded a journal called *Biometrica*. Today's journal editors might sympathize with the fact that in 1903, Pearson wrote to Galton that their journal had only two subscribers, both of whom were personal friends.

Greenwood staked his professional career on the claim that medical inference could be formalized by statistical methods. Greenwood exemplified Pearson's vision of the medical statistician as a hybrid social being, a researcher who understood both medical results and statistical methods. But medicine was slow to recognize the need for formal training in statistical methods. Greenwood criticized William Halstead, the famous Johns Hopkins surgeon, for failing to take age distribution into account when he reported statistics on the success of his surgery for cancer of the breast. "Surgeons in this country," he said, referring to the United States, "are mostly at the intellectual level of plumbers, in fact, [they are] just well-paid craftsmen." He continued, "I should like to shame them out of the comic opera performances which they suppose are statistics of operations and a really decent set of figures from such a panjandrum as Halstead would go a long way." Such was the acrimony that occurred during the struggle to create the milieu of the clinical trial as we know it today. By the 1960s, in the United States, the double-blind methodology had become mandatory for FDA approval, as it had in most other industrial democracies by the late 1970s.

Matthews expresses the idea that numerically presented results seem to have more authority whether they involve medical therapies, the outcome of elections or risk analysis. They are considered by some to represent objectivity and truth. He sees the emergence of the clinical trial as a special instance of a more general trend — the belief that numbers rule the world. Matthews asks these questions: "How much credence should be given to the professional expertise of the clinician and how much authority should be vested in the conclusions of the professional statistician? And how does the clinical trial fundamentally alter the nature of the doctor/patient relationship?" He asks one more very important question: "Do medicine's scientific credentials derive from the use of laboratory techniques or from mathematical statistical inference as used in epidemiology?" These questions are not new and were posed throughout the 19th and 20th centuries. Matthews reminds us that even today, what constitutes objectivity or science within medicine is still as hotly debated as it was in the Paris Academy of Medicine in 1837. With that in mind, Matthews ends his book with the French proverb, "Plus ça change, plus c'est la meme chose." The more things change, the more they stay the same.

Matthews' book, *Quantification and the Quest for Medical Certainty*, is well worth reading for its historical and philosophic perspectives on some of today's medical dilemmas and controversies. In a way, it's comforting to realize that while these issues may seem unique to our time, they're not actually new. The book has a further virtue — it's brief, with only 149 pages.

8

Streptomycin Treatment of Pulmonary Tuberculosis: The Classic Randomized Trial Turns 50

November 1998

The *British Medical Journal* of October 31, 1998 commemorates a landmark event, perhaps a watershed in the history of clinical medicine and research — "The Randomized Clinical Trial at 50." These words on the cover of the *BMJ*, along with a symbolic and not so subtle pair of dice, announce an issue devoted almost entirely to commentaries and reflections on the randomized clinical trial, which has become a paramount force in our clinical decisions and, with almost theatrical excitement, dominates much of today's clinical scientific meetings and journals. This theme issue marks the 50th anniversary of the publication in the *BMJ* on October 30, 1948, of a paper that is generally credited with introducing what might be called the randomized trial era. The paper, simply titled, "Streptomycin Treatment of Pulmonary Tuberculosis," was an investigation by the British Medical Research Council. One of the 15 members of the committee that planned the streptomycin for tuberculosis trial was Professor Austin Bradford Hill, now a legendary figure in the history of the randomized trial.

Among the 25 or so papers, editorials and commentaries devoted to various aspects of the randomized trial in this *BMJ* issue, one of the most comprehensive and insightful, I believe, is the one by Professor Richard Doll, an honorary member of the Clinical Trial and Epidemiological Studies Unit at the Radcliffe Infirmary in Oxford. Dr. Doll's career spans the modern era of clinical trials. He qualified for medicine in 1937 and was a student of Austin Bradford Hill. He recalls how at that time, new treatments were usually introduced by a professor or consultant at a leading teaching hospital who presented his clinical experiences with a few patients (rarely more than 50) who had been treated with a new method proclaimed to be more effective than that used by other clinicians or perhaps even his own earlier therapies. Obviously, this approach was not based on rigorous science or, in today's parlance, it was surely not evidence-based. As Dr. Doll points out, there were many claims of benefit. In 1948, he prepared a list of treatments for peptic ulcer disease so numerous that there was a treatment beginning with every letter of the alphabet.

Prior to 1948, there were sporadic efforts to find a more systematic method of comparing treatments, but none of them really solved the problem of bias. One approach was to alternate treatments depending on the day of hospital admission with placebos on one day and active agents on the other. But this method was vulnerable to bias because clinicians who preferred one treatment over another or who preferred a placebo, might stall admission until the appropriate day. This bias did occur, I believe, during the dicoumarol trials in the U.S. in the late 1940s, when alternate-day admissions for acute myocardial infarction were given dicoumarol or a placebo.

There was, however, one controlled clinical trial that antedated the landmark streptomycin for tuberculosis trial by 50 years — Johannes Fibiger's use of serum to treat diphtheria. Fibiger's trial is generally accepted as the first clinical trial in which random allocation was used successfully. Fibiger was a future Nobel Laureate. He wrote his doctoral thesis on diphtheria at the University of Copenhagen and was skeptical of the serum treatment for the disease. At age 28, he convinced his professor that a definitive trial was necessary, and in 1896 and 1897, he treated diphtheria patients either with twice-daily serum injections or with the standard treatment of the day which did not include serum. Allocation depended on the day of admission. Eight of the 239 patients in the serum group died compared with 30 of the 245 patients in the control group. There was no formal statistical analysis, but the effectiveness of serum was deemed obvious. In 1900, statistical methods appeared and a highly significant P-value was retrospectively determined for serum in the treatment of diphtheria.

I had never heard of Dr. Johannes Fibiger until I read the *BMJ* randomized trial issue. Later that same evening, after reading that issue of the *BMJ*, by chance I picked up an unread issue of *Perspectives in Biology and Medicine* that was more than a year old. My eye fell on an article called, "The Worm and the Tumor: Reflections on Fibiger's Nobel Prize." The name rang a bell and it turned out that this was indeed the same Fibiger of the diphtheria trial — how strange are the ways of serendipity. In the early 1900s, he found that a nematode worm was responsible for creating what he thought were cancers in the stomachs of wild rats. How he happened to be opening up the stomachs of wild rats was not mentioned, but shortly before his death in 1926, Fibiger received the Nobel Prize for this work. Unfortunately, it had been determined earlier by research in the United States that cancers were in fact not present in the rats. Thus, the work for which he received the Nobel Prize was invalid. The *Perspectives* article didn't mention Fibiger's work on diphtheria, now classic in the history of the randomized trial, but dwelled rather on the Nobel Prize given for spurious research.

In 1948, ethical committees didn't exist and no ethical criteria were laid down by the Medical Research Council (MRC) or anyone else. Medical ethics was defined by the Oath of Hippocrates, which every physician was required to take. The Medical Research Council in Britain had only a very small amount of streptomycin that they had purchased from the United States. Because it was not possible to treat the vast number of patients with tuberculosis who might benefit from streptomycin — which in the United States had been found to be effective in animals — the MRC chose to treat only inevitably fatal cases of miliary tuberculosis and meningitis. The small amount of streptomycin left over was used for the randomized trial. Patients who might have benefited from other treatments of the day — mainly those with pneumothorax — were excluded. Carefully matched patients with active TB were given streptomycin or allocated as controls. Placebos were not used because intramuscular injections of streptomycin were required four times a day. Random allocation in this trial removed any personal responsibility from clinicians who might have had bias either for or against streptomycin. The issue of patient consent was quickly dismissed with the question, "Does the doctor invariably seek a patient's consent before using a new drug alleged to be effective and safe?" If the answer were no, as it appeared to be at that time, there was no reason for a physician to seek permission to compare a new drug with an orthodox treatment.

As might have been expected, there was philosophic opposition to randomization. Sir Thomas Lewis, the British doyen of clinical research in the 1930s, rejected what he called "the statistical method of testing treatment." Lewis died in 1945, before randomized trials were introduced, but in his retrospective, Doll says that he could imagine what Lewis' reaction would have been. Lewis did believe that when testing treatments for acute diseases, two groups of similar patients should be treated concurrently in exactly the same way, except that one group should receive the remedy in question and the other should not. Lewis is quoted as saying: "It is to be recognized that the statistical method of testing treatment is never more than a temporary expedient and that little progress can come from it directly." Lewis objected to investigating cases collectively because there was still no way to determine which case would benefit and which would not. In answer to Lewis' objection, Bradford Hill remarked, "Tell me the criteria to distinguish patients who will respond from those who will not and we will build this into the trials." This problem persists today, because even though a significant number of patients may respond to a given intervention, all patients don't benefit. For this reason, in spite of our most sophisticated trials, we still have to treat many to help a few, not knowing which of the treated group will be helped.

Early randomized trials were criticized for being too small, but Doll recalls that Bradford Hill was trying to get a principle accepted and there were too few physicians, and especially surgeons, who were willing to expose their patients to cold scientific investigation. As a result, they had to be content with small trials. Trials such as ISIS were among the ones that inaugurated the modern era of huge international multicenter trials, which have become the order of the day. The streptomycin for TB trial had only 109 patients. Two died during the preliminary observation. Of the remaining 55, 107 were allocated to streptomycin and 50 to the control group. From the vantage point of today, it's interesting to look back at the specifics of this very small trial which had such a profound impact on the history of clinical research. The full text of this paper is available on the *British Medical Journal* website (http://www.bmj.com) along with an editorial titled, "The Control of Therapeutic Trials," by Austin Bradford Hill. This editorial takes pains to defend the use of an untreated control group, but argues that the effectiveness of streptomycin was still uncertain and finding out whether it was effective appeared to be the highest priority.

The lead editorial in the *BMJ* randomized trial issue is titled, "Unbiased Relevant and Reliable Assessments in Health Care: Important Progress During the Century, but Plenty of Scope for Doing Better." It is written by Ian Chalmers, Director of the U.K. Cochrane Center at Oxford. He considers the defining essence of the randomized trial to be the control of bias. Chalmers cites evidence that of the seven years of increased life expectancy achieved during the last half century, three years can be attributed to medical therapy, and much of the success and dissemination of medical treatment can be attributed to the randomized clinical trial. Chalmers warns against complacency and notes that in spite of thousands of randomized trials published since 1948, complete control of bias has not yet occurred.

Bias still exists today in the way randomized trials are interpreted and promulgated and in the way that samples are selected. These points are made in a paper titled, "Mammography and the Politics of Randomized Controlled Trials," also in the randomized trial issue of the

BMJ. In reviewing the history of randomized trials on screening mammography for breast cancer, this paper notes, for example, that the debate still continues today as to whether women under 50 should have periodic mammograms, and that conflicting advice and recommendations are still being given by professional and voluntary societies, doctors, journalists and research scientists. The paper makes it quite clear that political involvement and public expectations can and do impede appropriate translation of research findings into clinical practice.

In spite of massive numbers and sophisticated planning and statistics, randomized trials still don't provide monolithic consensus and clearly defined results. Bias may be controlled by perfecting randomized patient allocation, but it may still occur for a variety of ulterior reasons in dissemination and interpretation of results. These subjects are explored in some detail in yet another article in the *BMJ* commemorative issue, appropriately called, "Marketing Medicine Through Randomized Controlled Trials: The Case of Interferon."

In spite of the limitations of the randomized clinical trial, the importance of its contribution to the science of medical practice cannot be denied or minimized. Indeed, it is difficult to contemplate cardiology or medicine without the randomized trial. And even though it has turned 50 years old, or perhaps we should say 100, the randomized clinical trial remains both classic and contemporary.

9

Meta-Analysis Under Analysis

September 1997

An article in the August 21, 1997 issue of the *New England Journal of Medicine* entitled, "Discrepancies Between Meta-Analyses and Subsequent Large, Randomized, Controlled Trials" may be of great interest to all those who practice medicine and rely on the medical literature to help them make clinical decisions. It is written by Jacques LeLorier and his colleagues from the Hotel-Dieu Hospital and the Department of Medicine at the University of Montreal. The premise that led to this paper is that while large, randomized, controlled trials are generally considered the gold standard, these trials are not always available and, as a result, clinicians must often rely on meta-analyses to determine optimal clinical strategies.

In attempting to evaluate meta-analyses, the authors searched the *New England Journal of Medicine*, the *Lancet*, the *Annals of Internal Medicine*, and the *Journal of the American Medical Association* published between January 1, 1991 and December 31, 1994 for all randomized trials that involved 1000 patients or more. To achieve the specified objectives of their study, all of the trials had to have adequate statistical power. Then they sought meta-analyses on similar topics that had been published before the randomized trials in question. Each trial was matched with a corresponding meta-analysis, and only those that coincided with the trials in terms of population characteristics, therapeutic interventions and at least one target endpoint were selected. There were 12 randomized trials and 19 prior meta-analyses with 40 primary and secondary endpoints. The positive predictive value of the meta-analyses was 68 percent and the negative predictive value was 67 percent. If there had been no subsequent randomized trials, the meta-analyses would have led to errors or inappropriate treatment one-third of the time and to the rejection of errors or effective treatment also one-third of the time.

There are several reasons why a meta-analysis might have shown positive results that were not confirmed by a subsequent randomized trial. One of these is publication bias. There is a tendency for investigators to submit papers with positive results and a similar tendency for editors to accept them. Another reason is that even though the protocols of the trials selected in a meta-analysis study may look similar, there may be small differences in diagnostic criteria, coexisting conditions and severity of disease. These differences, which may not be readily apparent, can lead to differing results.

Considering that the comparison with randomized trials shows a poor predictive capacity, how then should clinicians use meta-analyses? There is probable agreement that a large, well-done, randomized trial should take precedence in medical decision-making and in practice guidelines, but if there is no such large trial and reliance must be made on several small randomized trials, then it seems that meta-analysis is the most simple, popular and attractive solution.

The Montreal study suggests that summarizing information in a set of trials with a single odds ratio may greatly oversimplify a very complex issue. Meta-analysis may be popular, at least in part, because it makes life easier for reviewers and readers. But this oversimplification may lead to erroneous conclusions. The authors, therefore, encourage readers to go beyond the aggregate findings of a meta-analysis and to look carefully at the studies that were included, particularly for consistency.

In this same issue of the *New England Journal*, there is an editorial entitled, "The Promise and Problems of Meta-Analysis," that critiques the Montreal paper and meta-analyses in general. The author, John Bailar of the University of Chicago, asks how the clinician should deal with the problem of a large, randomized, controlled trial that disagrees with a meta-analysis. Bailar, too, emphasizes the pitfalls of doing a valid meta-analysis. It usually requires close collaboration between clinicians and experienced statisticians. Investigators must try to find every relevant report by searching databases and bibliographies. Even unpublished work that has not been peer-reviewed may be included, and this may further compromise the reliability of a meta-analysis. The collected papers may have to be cut to less than 10 percent to meet the requirements for an effective meta-analysis. When the study is completed and submitted for publication, the editor and the reviewers should require from the authors rigorous technical analysis to identify, re-abstract and interpret a fair sample of the papers on which the meta-analysis is based. But Bailar thinks very few editors and reviewers will do this — and perhaps this is the reason there are so many poor meta-analyses in the literature.

Bailar contends that when both a randomized trial and a meta-analysis seem to be of good quality, he would tend to believe the results of the trial. The 40-year history of generally successful randomized, controlled trials has made important contributions that cannot be overlooked and neither can the many problems that may occur as a result of implementing a poorly done meta-analysis. It's not uncommon to find incompatible or even contradictory results in meta-analyses that were done at approximately the same time by investigators who had access to the same literature. Such disagreement argues powerfully against the notion that meta-analysis offers an assured way to distill the truth from a collection of research reports.

Bailar says that he knows of no instance in medicine where a meta-analysis, prior to a conventional review of the literature, has caused a major change in policy. Based on current evidence, Bailar believes that it may be acceptable to rely on a meta-analysis as a method of synthesizing the results of disparate studies on a common scale, but any attempt to reduce the results of even a well-done meta-analysis to a single value with confidence bounds is likely to lead to conclusions that are wrong and perhaps seriously so. He favors the conventional, familiar narrative review of the literature over meta-analysis.

Meta-analysis is not yet at a point where its findings can be considered sufficiently reliable when no confirmation is available and Bailar believes that that day is still well in the future. He agrees with the Montreal authors that even a large, randomized, controlled trial should be regarded more circumspectly than the published reports usually suggest. Finally, Bailar, somewhat cynically though perhaps correctly, believes that we never know as much as we think we know. Based on my experience, and I suspect that of most clinicians and investigators, Bailar's statement is true when it applies both to meta-analysis and to randomized, clinical trials.

In the September 6, 1997 issue of the *Lancet*, there is an editorial entitled, "Meta-Analysis Under Scrutiny" that explores the issue raised by the Montreal paper and its accompanying editorial. The *Lancet* editorial says that so far this year, it has received 34 meta-analyses or systematic reviews, but that, obviously, they can't use many of them. It also says that while these papers are not without problems — some are defective and some are duplications — there are plenty of homes for them such as the electronic media. The *Lancet* predicts that the *New England Journal* will receive many angry letters about the Montreal paper from systematic reviewers and authors of meta-analyses and that it will provoke debate on the place of quantitative meta-analysis in this era of mega-trials, but it doubts that meta-analysis can offer truth. While it does bring together unpublished and published trials as an aid to clinical judgment, meta-analysis now risks becoming a subspecialty unto itself, perhaps even an industry with its own jargon. The editorial also says that it's unfortunate that the *New England Journal* didn't publish a balancing editorial.

Just as I was about to conclude this editorial, the September 13, 1997 issue of the *British Medical Journal* arrived. On its cover, in bold print, is the headline, "Meta-Analysis: Separating the Good from the Bad." The journal includes an editorial trying to do just that and also several incisive papers. In an editorial entitled, "Meta-Analysis and the Meta-Epidemiology of Clinical Research," the author, David Naylor of Toronto, looks at the limits of meta-analysis but concludes, somewhat more optimistically than either the *New England Journal* articles or the *Lancet* editorial, that while meta-analysis continues to make contributions to medical research and to clinical decision-making, by the standards of medical reporting, it too is no panacea. It remains up to the reader to view each meta-analysis critically and to look particularly for heterogeneity in the clinical trials on which it reports. Naylor warns that if the process of pooling data inadvertently drowns out clinically important evidence from individual studies, then a meta-analysis can do more harm than good.

Turning back to the *Lancet* editorial, perhaps its most memorable comment is that a meta-analysis is valid only until the next good trial comes along. Finally, I'm reminded of an adage, the source of which I do not know, but it seems to apply — meta-analysis is to analysis as metaphysics is to physics.

10

Evidence-Based Medicine: A Clinical Critique

February 1999

The landmark paper, "Streptomycin Treatment for Pulmonary Tuberculosis," published in 1948 in the *British Medical Journal*, is generally considered to have marked the beginning of the randomized trial. It also signaled the coming ascendancy of evidence-based medicine (EBM) with the randomized trial as its centerpiece and gold standard. But even in the most sophisticated trials with massive numbers, absolutes are rare. Bias may not be completely controlled, randomization may not be perfect and the results are rarely without controversy. Also, marketing efforts often take liberties that end up having a major impact on the way results are interpreted and applied clinically. Nevertheless, the randomized trial is one of the single most important elements in today's medical and surgical decision-making. It is, perhaps, the sine qua non of what we like to think of as today's evidence-based medicine. To question or challenge even obliquely the primacy of EBM today is tantamount to "climbing Olympus in the face of the deity," a phrase that one of my teachers liked to use when questioning, as he often did, ideas and doctrines that seemed unassailable.

Something of the iconoclast comes through in a very thoughtful and elegantly written paper titled, "The Limitations of Evidence" in the Autumn 1998 issue of *Perspectives in Biology and Medicine*. The author, Sir Douglas Black, a former President of the Royal College of Physicians in England, agrees with Oxford's Dr. David Sackett, arguably the high priest of evidence-based medicine, who describes EBM as the conscientious, explicit and judicious use of the best evidence currently available for making decisions about the care of individual patients. Sackett adds that EBM can be described as the integration of individual clinical expertise with the best available evidence from systematic research. Dr. Black has no difficulty accepting this definition, particularly since it includes individual clinical expertise.

38

While Dr. Black supports the obvious virtues of evidence-based medicine, he does think it has some limitations, as the title of his paper suggests. Reminiscent of my teacher's allusion to climbing Olympus in the face of the deity, Dr. Black notes that "even to think of disparaging the evidence-based approach must be the cardinal sin of an academic physician." Black says that his backsliding began in a meeting convened to advise on the management of the permanent vegetative state which is not free from uncertainty, both in diagnosis and treatment. But during that meeting, the group was told that "all advice coming from the Department of Health must be evidence-based." Dr. Black responds, with some restraint I think, that "this was certainly a boldly stated idea, but scarcely corresponded to reality unless one stretches evidence to include the whole area in which we are guided by that illusive quality, 'common sense.'" In medicine, he adds, our concern is rarely with certitude but rather with the degree of probability needed to justify an action.

Dr. Black describes the randomized trial as a milestone in medical history, both in theory and in practice, and a brilliant response to the increasing proliferation of the highly effective, but potentially hazardous agents that we all use in practice. But his cardinal criticism of modern evidence-based medicine is the primacy given to the randomized trial over other sources of evidence that should go into the decision-making process. The most important derogation of the effectiveness of the randomized clinical trial, in Dr. Black's opinion, stems from patient variability and the wide spectrum of clinical syndromes that are often lumped under a single diagnostic category, such as nephrotic syndrome. In such instances, he contends that randomized trials may become inconclusive or conflicting, although they are probably still more effective than the results of unsystematized observations.

Dr. Black is also concerned that Sackett's "best available external clinical evidence" from systematic research may omit relevant evidence derived from many other sources, including the basic sciences, social sciences, epidemiology, natural history of disease and, not least of all, skill and diagnosis in which speaking with the patient is paramount. He fears that the inappropriate application of evidence not gained from the patient might be analogous to the old-fashioned danger of being sent to the wrong specialist. The current equivalent of this would be entering the patient into the wrong algorithm — one that would be more appropriate for another patient.

Dr. Black concludes that his purpose is not to disparage evidence-based medicine, but to deprecate any attempt to equate it to the totality of medicine. He also makes what I believe is an extremely important point — that when all of the evidence is gathered, the transition from knowledge to action may be based on evidence that was derived from comparable situations, but not necessarily from identical situations. Treatment requires continued intellectual review; without it, the errors that may occur can lead to preventable disasters in both individuals and groups.

In the *British Medical Journal* of January 30, 1999, a paper entitled, "Narrative-Based Medicine in an Evidence-Based World," by Trisha Greenhalgh of London, explores what Greenhalgh calls the dissonance between the science of objective measurement and the art of clinical proficiency and judgment. She notes that conventional medical training views medicine as a science and views the doctor as an impartial investigator who builds a differential diagnosis according to scientific theories. Greenhalgh contends that in the clinical encounter between doctor and patient, there is an interpretive act that requires what she calls "narrative skill" to integrate the overlapping stories told by the patient, the clinicians and the test results. She says the conflict between the science of objective medicine and the art of clinical proficiency and judgment occurs when the clinician only applies research findings to the clinical encounter and abandons the narrative and interpretive approach.

That scientific clinical evidence should underlie every medical decision is an ideal to be devoutly sought, but it is uncertainty rather than certainty that we are more likely to encounter. To impose the illusion of evidence-based certainty to the denigration of judgment, experience and common sense is not in the best interests of the patient, the doctor or society. The interpretation of evidence is not absolute, it is rarely universally agreed upon, and it is inevitably vulnerable to change. In his insightful article, Dr. Douglas Black also notes that the government — and I would add, other entities that finance and control medical care — may impose its interpretation of evidence for purposes other than the best interests of the patient.

For all these reasons, the papers that I have discussed here are important. They express valuable ideas and healthy skepticism as we try to blend the obvious virtues of evidence-based medicine with other sources of information and with the subtleties and the intuitive and subjective aspects of the doctor/patient encounter that cannot easily be reduced to absolutes and algorithms.

11

Guidelines and Intuition: Counterpoints in the Art of Medicine

May 1999

Among the many conflicts and contradictions encountered by doctors of today, perhaps none is more vexing than the demands for uniformity and conformity in practice on one hand and the historic role of the doctor to exercise judgment in the care of patients on the other.

During the past 25 to 30 years, several factors have, with geometric progression, increased scrutiny and control over decisions made in everyday practice. Important among these is the fact that widespread variations in medical practice occur among apparently similar patient populations in various geographic areas in the United States. Even more important is the progressive and now all-pervasive intrusion, both by government and the private sector, into virtually all aspects of the healthcare enterprise. With these developments have emerged guidelines, clinical pathways and a myriad of protocols and policies and, as an inevitable corollary, so too have the denigration and decline of respect for judgment and the art of medicine, once considered among the most important elements in effective practice.

While these forces appear to be exercising inexorable domination, there are voices of dissent. In the May 26, 1999 issue of the *Journal of the American Medical Association,* there is an article entitled, "Are Guidelines Following Guidelines? The Methodological Quality of Clinical Practice Guidelines in the Peer-Reviewed Medical Literature." The study, headed by Terrance Shaneyfelt from the University of Alabama in Birmingham, analyzes guidelines that were published in peer-reviewed journals to determine the degree to which they follow methodological standards that have been developed by organizations such as the Institute of Medicine and the American and Canadian Medical Associations, among others. Some 279 guidelines published between 1985 and 1997 were analyzed using a 25-item instrument. Their results showed that adherence to guidelines was generally weak

— overall averaging only 43 percent. The greatest need for improvement was in the identification, evaluation and synthesis of scientific evidence. Thus, guidelines themselves, important as they appear to be, are far from absolute. It seems that guidelines don't follow guidelines for guidelines very well.

In a somewhat critical accompanying editorial entitled, "The Trials and Tribulations of Clinical Practice Guidelines," Cook and Giacomini, from McMaster University in Hamilton, Ontario, found that "guideline developers must often reckon with research that is modest in rigor, discordant or nonexistent." They ask whether guidelines are written from the perspective of patients, practitioners, administrators, society or a combination. They emphasize that guidelines are indeed only guidelines and that they are intended to inform rather than tell us, with pious certitude, what to do. They also say that the guidelines may or may not use sources of wisdom other than research and that this may very well make guidelines more clinically useful. The authors concede that their study was not designed to measure various influences on guidelines, whether scientific, financial or editorial. But in spite of the guideline caveats alluded to in this editorial, guidelines are de facto standards, as anyone who has testified in a court of law knows very well. While those who write guidelines do offer the disclaimer that they are merely guidelines and nothing more, in reality they are much more.

As far back as 1993, Jerome Kassirer, editor of the *New England Journal of Medicine*, wrote an article entitled, "The Quality of Care and the Quality of Measuring It." In it, he asks whether the tools on which guidelines and appropriateness criteria are based are really valid and ready for widespread implementation. In essence, Kassirer asks the very same questions that were raised in the two above-mentioned papers from the May 26th issue of *JAMA*.

In the book, *Market Driven Healthcare: Who Wins, Who Loses in the Transformation of America's Largest Service Industry?* written in 1996 by Regina Hertzlinger, a professor at the Harvard School of Business with a special interest and a great deal of experience in healthcare, she describes a conflict in medicine between dogma and art. I don't think that in this context she is using the word dogma in a pejorative sense. But she certainly does imply that accepted dogma, including guidelines, is by no means immutable. She goes on to say that good doctors "are artists who must creatively fashion the diagnosis and therapy that best meets the needs of each individual patient."

What I've said thus far is perhaps an introduction to an intriguing article I came across in the Spring 1997 issue of *Perspectives in Biology and Medicine* entitled, "An Understanding of Intuition and Its Importance in Scientific Endeavor," written by Lois Eismann from the Department of Physiology at Tufts Medical School. Eismann begins by saying that when she asked scientific colleagues about the role of intuition in science, their answers ranged from "intuition is for poets, not for scientists" all the way to "it's all intuition." After asking what intuition really is, she then pursues several approaches to understanding the meaning of the word — and there are several. For example, when a physicist says that something is "intuitively evident," it means that it's obvious by inspection and doesn't require any further proof — in other words, it is something that is clear, straightforward and unchallenged. Sometimes the word intuition is used interchangeably with the word "instinct," which has quite another meaning. Intuition is also used to mean "a hunch," an idea that comes to mind without any idea of why and one that is not necessarily backed by data or fact. In this sense, the meaning of intuition is antithetical to the definition used by physicists for a thing so obvious it requires no further proof.

Intuition may also come from extensive knowledge that can be synthesized almost instantly. An example of this is when Linus Pauling first heard about the behavior of the red cell in sickle-cell anemia. With his extensive previous study of hemoglobin, he immediately predicted that the disease was caused by a simple genetic mutation that made hemoglobin aggregate at a low oxygen tension to distort and make rigid the red cell membrane. This use of the word intuition is in total contrast to "the hunch" or the "intuitive leap," in which a decision is made without hesitation, but wherein the intervening steps leading to the decision are not immediately apparent or accessible. Thus, an intuitive conclusion may be reached without awareness of the steps leading up to it. Further investigating the concept of intuition, Eismann reports that she was surprised when a colleague referred to intuition as something that occurred "in the blink of an eye." In this instance, an intuitive act occurs through unconscious processing involving analogies to other events and experiences. The concept is that intuition plays an important role in the process of scientific inquiry because of its access to unconscious content and its capacity for associative data management, both of which bring speed to creativity. Intuition can focus attention on circumstances or data that appear unrelated. Einstein referred to this capacity of intuition to uncover patterns in diverse phenomena when he said: "To these elementary laws there leads no logical path, but only intuition supported by being sympathetically in touch with experience." I believe these words apply equally to the process of clinical judgment and that many astute medical decisions, often the most difficult ones, do not follow logic or even a definable path, but occur by being sympathetically in touch with experience. And when Einstein used the word "experience," I presume he also meant knowledge.

In the September 1987 issue of *Science*, there is a paper titled, "The Cognitive Unconscious," by John Kihlstrom, that considers the idea that conscious perceptions may be the result of unconscious inferences based on knowledge and memory of past experiences. What we call intuition may result from a bridging function that somehow brings the cognitive unconscious into conscious thought. As Lois Eismann puts it, "through intuition, the unconscious, with its vast memory banks and accessing systems and the ability to process multiple items in parallel, may greatly enrich the capacities of the conscious mind, resulting in what we call intuition and at times permitting the intuitive leap."

While intuition cannot be quantified and defined in specific terms, it is a quality of vital importance in clinical medicine and it should not be cast aside entirely or subverted by rigid protocols and guidelines which themselves are far from absolute and often not applicable to a given patient or situation. In the 19th century, Peter Mere Latham said, "We have to cultivate a science and to exercise an art." Intuition and a successful intuitive leap (and, perhaps, even an unsuccessful one) may occur by the unconscious synthesis of science and art which, in medicine, finds expression as clinical judgment.

12

The Trouble with "Appropriateness"

November 1996

In the November 2, 1996 issue of the *Lancet,* there is an article that I believe will be of interest to all doctors who strive to define "appropriateness" in the practice of medicine. The article is entitled, "Are the Marginal Returns of Coronary Artery Surgery Smaller in High-Rate Areas?" by Janet Hux and David Naylor and the Steering Committee of the Provincial Adult Cardiac Network of Ontario. The observation that led to this study is that because rates of bypass surgery in a given population tend to vary within and between geographic areas, there is concern as to whether case selection may be less appropriate in the areas that have high rates of bypass surgery.

The authors point out, however, that appropriateness criteria generated by expert panels have not shown more inappropriate bypass surgery in high-rate areas and institutions. Therefore, they applied a "trial-based measure of projected survival benefit" for coronary bypass patients in the Ontario Provincial Registry to determine whether there was in fact a relationship between improved survival and rates of bypass surgery. The authors performed a retrospective review using linked registry and administrative data sets in some 5000 Ontario bypass patients between April 1, 1992 and March 31, 1993.

The Ontario study defined surgical appropriateness based on the results of randomized clinical trials as expressed by the coronary artery bypass graft surgery trialists collaboration published by the *Lancet* in 1994. There were unexplained variations in the rate of bypass surgery in the six cities and nine hospitals in Ontario that were doing bypass surgery and there were high bypass rates in three of the cities. The results show that overall, case selection was appropriate whether assessed clinically or on the basis of survival benefit scores. Clinical assessment was based on coronary artery anatomy with moderate to severe angina and by these criteria, 96 percent of bypass surgery was appropriate. Based on predicted moderate to high survival benefit scores, 94 percent were appropriate, but the proportion of projected low-benefit cases was greater in high-risk surgical centers.

In trying to understand the reason for the increased number of operations in patients with projected marginal benefits in the regions with high bypass rates, Hux and Naylor point out that appropriateness is not a straightforward designation. They cite the Rand Corporation's use of expert panels and the Delphi Method to judge appropriateness. When the Rand criteria were applied to coronary angiography, higher-rate regions did have higher proportions of inappropriate procedures, but the proportion that ranged from 15 to 18 percent was not sufficient to explain a two- to three-fold variation in the rates of angiography. The Rand consensus panel method has been criticized for subjectivity, bias, lack of precision in classifying appropriateness and inadequate statistical power.

It had been assumed that the rate of surgical procedures would be highly appropriate in areas where utilization was low and that as rates increased, there might be an increasing proportion of marginally appropriate or inappropriate cases. This was proved not to be the case by expert panel appropriateness criteria. Unlike analyses using consensus panel ratings, however, the Ontario study showed a definite and statistically significant negative correlation between bypass rate and projected survival benefit scores. In other words, as the rate of bypass surgery increased, more cases with marginal benefit were done.

The authors emphasize two differences between panel-based criteria and the projected benefit score calculated in the present study. Panel-based criteria define procedures by risk/benefit ratios as understood by a group of experts, but within the category of appropriate care, there will be a range of risk/benefit ratios. On the other hand, the trial-based approach used in the Ontario study permits assessment of the degree of potential survival benefit by bypass surgery in patients for whom the procedure would generally have been considered appropriate. The authors point out that in America — the world's most expensive and litigious healthcare system with by far the highest rates of cardiovascular procedures — any procedure "with even a minimally positive benefit/risk ratio may be affordable and defensible." But for nations with less affluent healthcare systems and far lower rates of bypass procedures, would marginal benefit cases be likely to occur more frequently as population-based rates rise? The answer, according to Hux and Naylor, is yes.

The authors suggest that the previous finding that rates are unrelated to appropriateness may be a "methodological chimera." Since you might, as I did, have some difficulty in understanding the use of the term chimera in this context, I looked it up in Webster's dictionary and found that in addition to the she-monster of Greek mythology, chimera can also mean "an illusion or fabrication of the mind or fancy, or a utopian or unrealizable dream or aim." Perhaps it's not a bad choice of a word to describe the problem of defining appropriateness.

Hux and Naylor's provocative paper seems logically to lead to further consideration of the status and limitations of our ability to define appropriateness and evidence-based medicine in general. David Naylor has a thoughtful essay in the April 1995 issue of the *Lancet*, titled, "Gray Zones in Clinical Medicine: Limits to Evidence-based Medicine." He refers to a 1993 *New England Journal* article by Sandra Tannenbaum of Ohio State University, titled, "What Physicians Know." Of Tannenbaum's paper, Naylor says: "In a recent attack on evidence-based medicine, a philosopher urged doctors to defend clinical reasoning based on experience and pathophysiological mechanisms and criticized the effects of clinical epidemiology and health services research on practice." While Naylor says he wishes that the effects of epidemiology and health services research were more pervasive, he does concede that a backlash is not surprising in view of inflated expectations from outcomes-oriented and evidence-based medicine and the fears of some clinicians that these concepts may threaten the art of patient care.

Naylor believes that evidence-based medicine offers little help in the gray zones of practice where the evidence about risk/benefit ratios for completing clinical options is incomplete and contradictory. So-called expert panels use not only evidence, but also inference and experience and consequently, they may be pooling ignorance as much as distilling wisdom. Naylor somewhat cynically observes that in trying to marshal expert consensus, clinical guideline writers may fail to distinguish fact from fervor. Naylor closes his essay by paraphrasing Sir William Osler, saying that good clinical medicine will always be a blend of the art of uncertainty and the science of probability.

In a 1994 paper in the *British Medical Journal*, "Some Observations on Attempts to Measure Appropriateness of Care," N.R. Hicks of Oxford cites an increasing number of studies suggesting that healthcare is often delivered inappropriately. In this very interesting and thought-provoking paper, Hicks explores the assumptions inherent in currently available measures of appropriateness and their impact on practice. Hicks summarizes his views by saying that although appropriateness guidelines may seem to be objective and systematic, the process by which they are produced remains highly subjective. He makes what I think is a very cogent point — that measures of appropriateness are really not sufficiently robust to be used with confidence to influence or control the delivery of healthcare and that appropriateness studies may be better used as an aid than as a constraint in clinical decision-making. Finally, Hicks proposes the inevitable — a randomized clinical trial that he thinks could resolve the question of whether patients receive better outcomes if their care is influenced by appropriateness criteria. His proposal is, I think, fanciful at best, considering the uncertain status of appropriateness criteria — even without considering the question of whose criteria are really appropriate enough to randomize.

13

The Tyranny of "Value-Neutral Cold Statistics" in Government and Medicine

December 1995

As we approach the year's end, or perhaps to put it more dramatically, as we are about to enter the last half of the last decade of the 20th century, it might be well to look beyond medicine for some perspective on our profession and our role in it.

Last October, while vacationing in Florida, I was browsing through the Autumn 1995 edition of the *Wilson Quarterly* when I came upon the review of a book called *The Tyranny of Numbers: Mismeasurement and Misrule*. This most fascinating book is written by Nicholas Eberstadt, a demographer by training, a visiting fellow at the Harvard Center for Population and Development Studies and a visiting scholar at the American Enterprise Institute for Public Policy Research. I don't suppose there is any thoughtful practicing or academic doctor who wouldn't think that somehow, somewhere in a book on the tyranny of numbers there might be an application, or at least an analogy to the medicine of today.

The foreword of Eberstadt's book is written with characteristic insight and wit by Senator Patrick Moynihan of New York. Moynihan recalls that somewhere in the writings of George Orwell, there is an account of a rumor that during World War II, when American troops arrived in Britain, they were not there to invade the continent, but to put down an incipient workers' revolt in the British war industries, perhaps reminiscent of Petrograd in 1917. Orwell observed that to believe such an absurdity, you would have had to have gone to a university and that even a London cab driver could have told you it was nonsense.

To illustrate the occasional fallacy of numbers, Eberstadt cites the 1989 edition of *Statistical Abstracts of the United States*, a Bureau of the Census publication that draws on data from various governmental agencies, including the Central Intelligence Agency. The *Statistical Abstracts* include an estimate of the economies of East and West Germany and came to the conclusion that the 1985 per capita output of East Germany was equal to that of West Germany and perhaps even slightly higher. These data, as Eberstadt explains, came from an unclassified and widely circulated CIA publication. But as Senator Moynihan notes, any Berlin taxi driver crossing over Check Point Charlie can tell you that the economy of West Germany was vastly superior to that of East Germany. Moynihan refers to Nicholas Eberstadt as our taxi driver in spotting the fallacies in statistics by which our government sets much of its policy.

Moynihan quotes Eberstadt's observation that once statistics are invested with political powers, they can injure human beings. Modern governments, rationalist and problem-solving as they are in orientation, imbue statistics with political power by using them to set their policies. The power accorded to these mute and inanimate numbers is far-reaching. Under modern governance, the impetus for state action typically extends well beyond the limits of knowledge that available data are providing — or indeed, could ever possibly provide. This, according to Eberstadt, is the perilous terrain over which the tyranny of numbers prevails.

Eberstadt has a considerable facility for turning a phrase. One that particularly appeals to me is this: "Where antique despots surrendered to the temptations of numerology, the modern statesman proudly succumbs to the allure of 'quantophrenia,'" a term he didn't invent, but by which he means "an idolatry of numbers no less unreasoning and no less poorly suited for promoting the commonwealth, than its precursor — that is numerology." The fundamental thesis in Eberstadt's collection of essays is that the consequences are injurious when a problem-solving government uses inaccurate data, selects accurate but inappropriate indicators or misanalyzes available facts and figures.

The *Tyranny of Numbers* was also reviewed in the December 1995 issue of *Commentary*. This review emphasizes one of the few medically related discussions in Eberstadt's book. It concerns the cited infant mortality rate in the United States, which, because it is high by international standards, is often used as an indictment against American medicine. It is often invoked as evidence that the U.S. healthcare system is a failure, and it points to a need for greater government involvement in healthcare. But Eberstadt's interpretation of the data refutes this idea. He suggests that the high infant mortality rate is misleading; the crucial cause, he believes, is not the inaccessibility of medical services, but rather, the personal behavior of women during pregnancy. He points out that the American medical system outperforms its foreign counterparts in treating low-birth-weight babies but that our society is unable to keep pregnant women from engaging in high-risk activities. Thus, the statistical data of high infant mortality may be accurate but the manner in which those data are interpreted is irrelevant, and our government continues this fallacy lest the victims — pregnant women — be blamed. Eberstadt argues further that misuse of statistical data — such as mislabeling various population problems — has hampered international efforts to deal more effectively with problems of malnutrition and economic distress, thereby diverting aid from where it is needed most.

It is an unfortunate reality that value-neutral cold statistics are used to drive policy, even with regard to moral issues — and there is no substitute for moral reasoning in human affairs. Eberstadt concedes that the statistics-oriented ameliorative state may be new, but the question of how to use knowledge in a morally responsible way is not. If one substitutes the words clinical judgment where Eberstadt uses moral reasoning, the analogy to medicine becomes apparent. If we substitute the word medicine where Eberstadt refers to government, the analogy will be even clearer. In medicine, we are more and more governed by policies derived from statistics. This tendency applies to all spheres of medicine — education, science and practice — but especially to regulation by government and managed care organizations. Any patient or doctor having much contact with managed care will readily understand what Eberstadt means by "value-neutral cold statistics."

Our medical decisions do depend in large measure on statistics and their interpretation and this is true in all fields of medicine. Examples in cardiology are legion. They include lipid management, the use of ACE inhibitors and calcium channel blockers, and issues such as whether angioplasty or thrombolysis may be superior in acute myocardial infarction, whether angiography should or should not be performed in almost all patients following acute myocardial infarction, and even whether stents are the wave of the future or merely potential obstructions placed in coronary arteries. In sorting out clinical dilemmas, regardless of specialty or type of practice, the emphasis is on statistics. In the complex world of today's medicine, statistics are vital in understanding what we are doing and what we should be doing. Many of us are seduced by the tyranny of numbers, while others find so-called value-neutral cold statistics forced upon them.

In his companion editorial to an article in the *New England Journal of Medicine* on November 16, 1995, on the prevention of coronary heart disease with pravastatin in Scottish men with hypercholes-terolemia, T.R. Pedersen offers a sobering thought. In spite of the now incontrovertible evidence for the great value of reducing cholesterol, 215 subjects of the pravastatin group had coronary events in spite of a 26 percent reduction in low-density lipoproteins (LDLs). Pedersen re-minds us further that in the Scandinavian Simvastatin Survival Study (known as the 4S study) with a 35 percent reduction in LDL choles-terol, one-fifth of the treated group still had new coronary events. In the widely publicized and perhaps landmark West of Scotland Study (WOSCOPS), the five-year death rate from all cardiac causes was re-duced by only 0.7 percent between the placebo and pravastatin cohorts of some 3300 patients each.

As Eberstadt suggests, value-neutral cold statistics may drive pol-icy, but moral issues (and I might add, clinical judgments) cannot to-tally be subordinated to them. Perhaps what we really need is one of Senator Moynihan's down-to-earth, commonsense London or Berlin cab drivers. Eberstadt believes that when the novelty of what he calls the "Probabilistic Revolution" begins to fade, it will be recognized around the world that governmental policy determined by statistics is policy based on potentially flawed interpretations that may be injurious to both present and future generations. This philosophy applies equally to medicine. In the present medical climate, a self-serving interpreta-tion of self-generated statistics by third parties and medical entrepre-neurs has unfortunately become a dominant force that adversely affects patients and their access to medical care.

14

Epidemiology at Risk? Or is It the Public?

August 1995

Augst should be a quiet time, a month of transition as summer begins to fade and vacations offer a respite even while the intensity of the new season looms just ahead. August, then, may be the right time to look beyond the medical literature and to see what those in the world outside of medicine are saying about some things medical.

On the cover of the August 1995 issue of *Forbes* magazine, there is a bold headline that trumpets, "How Business, Doctors and Journalists Prey on Your Food Anxieties." There is also a picture of a table set with a cup of coffee in which the outline of a skull can be seen. The cover story is entitled, "Lies, Damned Lies and Medical Statistics" and underneath, it says, "Doctors, journalists and health food vendors have us scared to death about what we eat, drink and breathe. But most of their studies couldn't pass Statistics 101." The article begins by mentioning the 1973 movie, *Sleeper*, in which Woody Allen portrays a health food salesman who awakens from suspended animation in the year 2173, asking for wheat germ, organic honey and Tiger's Milk. A puzzled 22nd-century doctor wonders why people once had preferred such "sludge" to steak, cream pies and hot fudge. His medical colleague answers, "Those foods were thought to be unhealthy; precisely the opposite of what we know to be true." The article continues: "Life imitates art and intimates that 20 years too late, we now learn that once highly touted margarine has transfatty acids worse for our arteries than any found in nature."

This somewhat tongue-in-cheek article proceeds with a litany of dangers by which we are bombarded through reports taken from the medical press. The author says that in spite of mercury-laden fish, coffee, eggs, chlorine and second-hand smoke, we seem to be living longer, healthier and better nourished lives than ever before. He describes the dilemmas faced by a public beset with contradictory information — on alcohol, for example. A *New England Journal of Medicine* editorial endorses the favorable effect of a daily drink on coronary disease and this contrasts with a more recent *New England Journal* paper telling how alcohol in large amounts can raise blood pressure. In the public press, the fine distinction between a little alcohol and a lot becomes lost or, at best, blurred.

One study that received wide publicity and was later discounted concerns the relationship between high-tension electric wires and cancer clusters. Another study, reported on the front page of the *Washington Post*, is one from 1991 from the University of British Columbia and California State at San Bernardino that left-handed people have shorter lives. Even though this latter report was later debunked in the *British Medical Journal* and in the *American Journal of Public Health*, the *Washington Post* story was never retracted.

In spite of the encouraging observation that our life expectancy in 1900 was 47 years and now it's 76 years, Americans continue to be bedeviled by the fear of dangers lurking in our environment. So pervasive is this fear that the fall 1990 issue of *Daedalus*, the journal of the American Academy of Arts and Sciences, was devoted entirely to the concept of risk. In that issue, Harvey Sapulski, Professor of Public Policy at MIT, commented that "hardly anyone is saved by the collective mania with risk. Many may be harmed by what goes undone. Scientists offer little solace in the quest for safety; on the contrary they often stoke public fears with their ever-increasing ability to detect low levels of potentially dangerous elements in commonly used products."

"In Search of Zero Risk" is the intriguing title of a February 1995 article in the *Wall Street Journal* that recalls the Thanksgiving season of 1989 when trace residues of a cancer-causing herbicide were found in cranberries, causing the U.S. Department of Health and Human Services to recommend against buying cranberries. This set off a panic that nearly devastated the cranberry industry. The article also recalls that back in the 1950s, the Eisenhower administration asked the National Cancer Institute to establish safe levels for cancer-causing substances, leading to the so-called one-in-a-million standard acceptable risk from environmental contaminants, intended to define a level beyond which regulation is inefficient. But the author of the article could find no one to give a scientific basis for this one-in-a-million standard. The article suggests that cleaning up all hazardous waste sites to a one-in-a-million level is in some ways comparable to reducing the highway speed limit to one mile an hour. The risks of speeding would be virtually eliminated, but getting to one's destination would be costly and painfully slow.

The *Wall Street Journal* is not alone in its criticism of observational epidemiological studies. More than a decade ago, in a *New England*

Journal of Medicine article entitled, "Double Standards, Scientific Methods and Epidemiological Research," Alvin Feinstein of Yale points out that the cohort and case control studies commonly used in epidemiology need to be performed and evaluated according to the same standards used in other branches of science.

In the July 14, 1995 issue of *Science,* a special report called, "Epidemiology Faces Its Limits," states that the search for subtle links between diet, lifestyle, environmental factors and disease is an unending source of fear that yields little certainty. In a more scientific way, this article offers exactly the same message as the August *Forbes* cover story. The *Science* article has a familiar theme — news about health risks comes thick and fast these days and seems almost constitutionally contradictory. One example is a January 1994 Swedish study claiming a relationship between residential radon and cancer and the subsequent refutation of this claim by a Canadian study. Other reports noted by *Science* that were later contradicted include the relationship between abortions and breast cancer and between electromagnetic fields from power lines and breast cancer and leukemia.

A 1994 *New England Journal* editorial asks, "What Should the Public Believe?" The authors, Drs. Angell and Kassirer, said "that health-conscious Americans increasingly find themselves beset by contradictory advice. No sooner do they learn the results of one research study than they hear a contradictory result." While Angell and Kassirer blame the press for the way it reports epidemiological studies and blame the public for its unrealistic expectations, their own distinguished publication, the *New England Journal,* is one of the foremost purveyors of the kind of epidemiological material that receives great attention in the nonmedical press.

Dimitrios Trichopoulos, an epidemiologist at the Harvard School of Public Health, is quoted in *Science* as saying that epidemiology is stretched to its limits and beyond. He notes that epidemiologists are fast becoming a public nuisance and people don't take them seriously any more. But he does suggest a solution. The press should be more skeptical of epidemiological findings and epidemiologists themselves should become more skeptical of their own work. Trichopoulos' observations recall a comment made several years ago in the *London Daily Independent* that America is a society drunk not on alcohol, but on random factlets wrested from the scientific journals before the ink is dry.

Norman Breslow of the University of Washington in Seattle says in *Science* that statistical significance — that is, a 95 percent confidence level — may mean considerably less than it seems to. It may ignore systematic errors, biases and other confounders. Sir Richard Doll, a famous epidemiologist and statistician at Oxford, who once co-authored a study erroneously suggesting that women who took reserpine had up to a fourfold increase of risk for breast cancer, suggests that no single epidemiological study is persuasive unless it defines at least a threefold increase in risk. Some prefer a fourfold risk. The rule of thumb at the *New England Journal* is a relative risk of 3 or more before accepting a paper for publication, particularly if it's biologically implausible or if it's a new finding. Others say a risk of 10 percent or more might be believed if it shows up consistently in different studies. Yet the article in *Science* catalogues some 25 articles purporting to relate various foods and exposures to different forms of cancer in which the risk ratio is well under 3 — most under 1.5 — and these articles were published in major peer-reviewed scientific journals. All or most of these scientific papers make their way into the public press without full explanation of the questionable nature of the risk — and follow-ups and retractions in the public press are rare.

Several years ago in *Dayton Medicine*, I wrote an article called, "At Risk at Breakfast on Thursday Morning." Thursday morning was a critical time because some of our leading weekly scientific medical journals embargo their material until 6 o'clock on Wednesday evening, just in time for the evening news and for Thursday morning's headlines. The one that caught my attention and led to that article was a lay press headline: "Coffee Harmless Study Finds — As Long As It's Not Decaf." This press report describes — without criticism — an article in one of our major medical journals.

The problem may lie not only in some inherent limitations of epidemiological research, but also, at least in part, in seductive press releases by our own scientific journals. These releases, perhaps unintentionally, tend to entice the lay press to premature and uncritical reporting to a public obsessed with the idea that life should be risk-free and that modern medicine can define and protect against every possible hazard. Perhaps William James had the best antidote for the health hazard of the week:

> It is only by risking our persons from one
> hour to another that we live at all.
> And often our faith beforehand in an
> uncertified result is the only thing
> that makes that result come true.

15

Medicine Between Two Worlds:
Modern and Post-Modern

January 1995

In the special annual year-end edition of the *British Medical Journal*, there is an article entitled, "Medicine at the Center of the Nation's Affairs: Doctors and Their Institutions are Failing to Adapt to the Modern World," by Sir Maurice Shock, former Rector of Lincoln College at Oxford. I would respectfully like to suggest to Sir Maurice that it is really the "post-modern world" to which doctors and their institutions are failing to adapt. Bruce Charlton of the Medical School at the University of Newcastle deals with this issue in a paper he wrote called, "Medicine and Post-Modernity," published by the Royal Society of Medicine in 1993. Charlton says that even though "post-modernism" is a rather pretentious way to describe what is happening in contemporary western society, it is a useful term.

The world of modernity and the modernist view of life began in the 17th century with Isaac Newton in science and René Descartes in philosophy and culminated in the 18th-century Enlightenment. The modernist point of view assumes that when rational people use diligent study and scientific methods, they can reach objectively definable truth. According to Enlightenment thinking, this applies to science, politics, morals — indeed, to all aspects of human endeavor.

Medicine is perhaps the quintessential example of modernity in that it relies on the accumulation of objective scientific knowledge to establish scientific truth. The ultimate symbol of modernity in medicine is the prospective randomized clinical trial which seeks to establish a standard for practice — or, in medical parlance, truth, at least truth in terms of what is known at a given time and what can be validated by rational inquiry. Medical modernity is also reflected in the view that only experts armed with evidence obtained by scientific inquiry are qualified to speak on technical medical matters. In contrast, the post-modern world is dominated by subjectivity in which rigidly defined scientific and medical concepts are merely expressions of professional authority assumed by scientists and doctors. Cultural relativism is the hallmark of post-modern philosophy. There are no absolutes and no unassailable truths; only subjective impressions and interpretations. This is obviously an oversimplification, but the essence of post-modernist thinking is that "truth" is refracted by the eye of the beholder. In contrast to the modernist view of truth as something that can be discovered and established, post-modernity favors relativism and individual preference.

Pauline Vaillancourt Rosenau, of the University of Texas Health Science Center in Houston, discusses this subject in a paper entitled, "Health Politics Meets Post-Modernism: Its Meaning and Implication for Community Organizing," in the Summer 1994 issue of the *Journal of Health Politics, Policy and Law*, published by Duke University Press. Rosenau points out that post-modernism does not necessarily reject reason and science but contends that reason and science are not necessarily superior to emotion and intuition. Thus, post-modern guidelines for healthcare would be created not only by experts such as specialist physicians, but also by nurses, technicians, patients, ethicists, behavioral scientists and other generalists. Post-modernism questions the authority of physicians and the assumption that medical science is a discipline with special privilege, knowledge and methodologies. To the post-modernist, medical objectivity is often a form of veiled self-interest.

Charlton believes that glimmerings of post-modern medicine are beginning to be seen in the United States "with medicine quietly abandoning science which is altogether too crude and inflexible to encompass the plurality of human pleasure and preference." He visualizes an abundance of alternative therapies that promise to enhance the consumer's lifestyle and sense of worth. In post-modern medicine, standards tend to be fluid, more personal and aesthetic. Distinctions between expert and consumer and physician and patient become blurred. Disease and illness would merge with health and well-being. In short, sickness is modern, while health is post-modern.

As long as medicine is dealing with sickness, modernity is preferable to post-modernity. When we are sick, we want to know that there is a reasonable expectation that our treatment is based on evidence that it will be effective. We want the assurance of proper professional science and ethics, not the cut and thrust (to use Charlton's words) of the marketplace. Economic efficiency must not be the primary aim; it should be subordinated to clinical goals. In other words, a sick person wants the certainties of modernity insofar as they are available. Only when we are feeling well are we inclined to gamble on the glamorous relativities of post-modernity.

Charlton quite astutely sees post-modern attitudes and practices dominating politics, philosophy, morals and art, but he finds strongly modernist practices persisting in medicine. Thus he sees contemporary medicine as an island of modernity floating in a shifting sea of post-modernity. Modernists give special authority to experts and believe in the positive role of high technology. Post-modernists believe that confidence in experts and new technology is sometimes misplaced.

A comparison of modernity, with its Enlightenment ideals and its reliance on the ultimate triumph of science, with the more subjective, and in some ways cynical, concepts of post-modernity, may seem arcane and remote from those of us in medicine. But understanding the implications of the modern and the post-modern viewpoint will help us to more successfully cope with the dilemmas and confrontations that the world of medicine faces today.

16

Alternative Medicine: A Flight from Science and Reason

October 1998

In the September 17, 1998 issue of the *New England Journal of Medicine*, editors Marcia Angell and Jerome Kassirer wrote an article called, "Alternative Medicine: The Risks of Untested and Unregulated Remedies." They define alternative medicine as a heterogeneous group of theories and practices that range from homeopathy to therapeutic touch to herbal medicine. In a 1993 *New England Journal* article entitled, "Unconventional Medicine in the United States," senior author David Isenberg, from Beth Israel Hospital in Boston, defines alternative medicine as "medical interventions not widely taught in U.S. medical schools or generally available in U.S. hospitals." But this definition is probably no longer valid because many alternative treatments have recently been accepted by medical schools, hospitals and HMOs, and some states even require that health plans cover alternative medical practices. As examples of alternative medicine, the Isenberg article cites acupuncture, chiropractic and massage therapy.

Angell and Kassirer believe that what sets alternative medicine apart is that it is not scientifically tested. Its advocates generally reject the need for such testing, contending that scientific method is really not applicable to their remedies. The influence of alternative medicine is so great that in 1992, the Congress established an Office of Alternative Medicine to evaluate such remedies within the National Institutes of Health. So far, the results have been disappointing. Since 1993, among 30 such grants by the NIH, there are 28 final reports, some of which are abstracts, listed in the NIH alternative medicine database. However, a Medline search reveals only nine published papers, five of which are in journals that are not generally recognized and the other four are uncontrolled clinical trials.

The thrust of the Angell and Kassirer editorial is that it is time for the scientific community to stop giving alternative medicine a free ride. Assertions, speculations and testimonials are no substitute for rigorous evidence of efficacy. The editorial calls for alternative treatments to be subjected to the same scientific testing required for conventional treatments. Angell and Kassirer see the increased interest in alternative medicine as a regression to the irrational at a time when scientific medicine is making its most dramatic advances. While decrying this paradox, they concede that the reasons for this trend are beyond the scope of their observations. They do, however, suggest the possibility that the rise of alternative medicine may be caused by the hurried and impersonal care often given by conventional doctors and by the harshness of some of the treatments used for life-threatening diseases. Unfortunately, this explanation seems inadequate and quite superficial.

A most intriguing book, published in 1996 by the New York Academy of Sciences, frames a much broader picture of alternative medicine than just a flight from and a rejection of scientific medicine. Instead, it points to a serious societal problem, aptly described in the title of the book: *The Flight from Science and Reason*. In a chapter titled, "Medicine Took an Earlier Flight," Henry Greenberg of New York's St. Luke's-Roosevelt Hospital, refers to recent assaults on medical professionalism, medical specialists and academic medicine and points to a widespread and pervasive trend in our society to invalidate scientific reasoning not only in medicine, but in all spheres. In the introduction to this book, P.R. Gross, from the Center for Cell Signaling at the University of Virginia, Charlottesville, reminds us that the flight from science goes back as far as science itself and really began in earnest with the 18th-century Enlightenment. He catalogues various forms of anti-reason and anti-science, many of which are still active today, including the cults of UFO watchers, the supposed victims of abduction by extraterrestrials, adjusters of human energy fields, and especially, the archaic mountebank healers and dispensers of potions. Gross notes that the rejection of reason occurs not only in scientific disciplines, but in most other areas of scholarship as well, including the humanities, religion, social sciences and health.

The authors of the article "Unconventional Medicine in the United States," mentioned earlier in this editorial, looked at the frequency of alternative treatments and concluded from their 1990 survey of a national sample of adults who were 18 years of age or older, that 34 percent had used at least one form of alternative therapy during the past year and that a third of those averaged 19 such therapies. Extrapolation to the U.S. population suggests that in 1990, Americans made 425 million visits to unconventional therapists as compared to 388 million visits to primary care doctors. Expenditures for alternative medicine in 1990 amounted to $13.7 billion, $10 billion of which was paid out of pocket, compared with $12.8 billion paid out of pocket for all hospitalizations in the United States. These figures exceed what had been thought to be the extent of alternative medicine expenditures in this country.

In his chapter in the New York Academy volume, "Anti-science Trends in the Rise of the Alternative Medicine Movement," Dr. Wallace Sampson of Stanford University School of Medicine points out that propaganda, cultural relativism and other post-modern doctrines that challenge objectivity are integral to today's unscientific thinking. He believes they are linked to a cabal of thought that is slowly strangling medical science. He believes that cultural relativism and post-modernism's rejection of objectivity are responsible for a good deal of today's medical mischief, such as the vogue for Laetrile as a cancer treatment a few years ago and the NIH's creation of an office for alternative medicine. To Sampson, post-modernism is an abstract and esoteric phenomenon that takes cultural relativism one step further into a disorienting world with no standards for accuracy or ethics. Alternative medicine, a product of post-modernism, puts relativism and value-free analysis above rigorously acquired scientific data.

Sampson quotes from a 1995 editorial by L. Dossey in the journal, *Alternative Therapies*, in which Dossey claims that many alternative interventions are different from surgical procedures and drugs because their actions are affected by factors that cannot be specified, quantified or controlled in double-blind designs. To subject alternative therapies to sterile, impersonal double-blind conditions, he adds, strips them of the intrinsic qualities that are part of their power. Dossey maintains that there are ineffable qualities inherent in alternative therapies that conventional methods cannot detect or define. His conclusion, therefore, is that alternative methods must be accepted, their practitioners licensed and their services paid for by public funds and health insurance.

If ever there was a visible flight from science and reason, it is to be found in the rapid shift — now manifest, to some extent, even within the healing professions themselves — from the rejection of quackery, to acquiescence, and finally to accommodation. As P.R. Gross notes in the introduction to the New York Academy volume, a few years ago, only *Saturday Night Live* would have featured a shaman gesturing above the head of a patient in open heart surgery. But today, this kind of spectacle may actually be found in one of our great university hospitals.

The New York Academy book, *The Flight from Science and Reason*, puts alternative medicine in the social context of our times. The assault by post-modernism is by no means confined to medicine, but poses a threat to all disciplines, from the hard sciences to the social sciences and to the humanities. In his chapter, "Flights of Fancy: Science, Reason and Common Sense," Barry Gross, editor of the book and a philosophy professor at the City University of New York, concludes by saying that we must make no mistake about what it will take to show up anti-science Luddites for what they are and to defeat them. And these two tasks — showing them up and defeating them — are by no means the same. Both will take organized, continuous, strong and clear opposition. We in medicine should heed this advice and take seriously the challenge that alternative medicine poses to the scientific, intellectual and ethical basis of our profession. I can't resist observing that much of the philosophy and much of what we object to in the managed care approach to medicine appears to be quite consistent with the ideas and concepts of post-modernism.

As a prelude to his incisive introduction to *The Flight from Science and Reason*, P.R. Gross quotes from Goethe's *Faust*. Mephistopheles, disguised in Faust's academic robes, is ready to receive a fawning student whom Faust had refused to see, and he whispers to Faust as he retreats from the room:

> Scoff at all knowledge and despise
> reason and science, those flowers of mankind.
> Let the father of all lies
> with dazzling necromancy make you blind,
> then I'll have you unconditionally.

It seems all too apparent that Goethe's Mephistopheles lives on, and as he predicted, holds all too many unconditionally.

17

The Clinton Plan and American Healthcare in Transition

April 1993

A nyone who doubts that the election of President Bill Clinton will result in major changes in healthcare must be out of touch. Perhaps no issue related to medicine has ever so dominated the political scene as that of healthcare reform. I am often asked what the College is doing with regard to the Clinton healthcare initiatives. The answer is that the College is monitoring the Clinton Task Force as closely as possible, although as you are well aware, little information is available on what is planned or how it is being planned. Only under intense pressure from the media, including the *New York Times*, the *Washington Post* and the national news magazines, and in response to legal action, has the Clinton healthcare plan been opened up at all.

In January 1993, Dolph Hutter, then President of the College, met briefly with the Clinton transition team. In February, Marie Michnich, Associate Executive Vice President for Health Policy, attended a White House briefing with Domestic Affairs Advisor Ira Magaziner. The College was well represented at the March 24, 1993 AMA meeting in Washington, called, "A Time for Partnership," at which the AMA demanded a voice in healthcare reform. I attended that meeting as President of the College, along with Dolph Hutter, immediate past President; Dan Ullyot, President-Elect; Bill Marshall, Chairman of the ACC Government Relations Committee, and Marie Michnich and Karen Collishaw of the Health Policy Department. Top leaders on both sides of the aisle addressed the meeting, including Vice President Gore, Senate Majority Leader George Mitchell and Minority Leader Robert Dole. If there was consensus, it was that the role of the physician is vital and that our voice will be heard. But the Democrats, including Senators Rockefeller and Kennedy, Congressman Pete Stark and Health and Human Services Secretary Shalala, gave no inkling of what the Clinton Task Force has in mind. The Republicans, especially Senator Phil Gramm of Texas and Newt Gingrich, Minority House Whip from

Georgia, made it clear that any healthcare bill will be subjected to full discussion in the Congress. In support of that idea from the other side of the aisle, House Majority Leader Richard Gebhart, who did not attend the AMA meeting but spoke afterward, said, "we're going to take our time, we're going to listen to the American people."

On March 26th, two days after the AMA meeting, Marie Michnich and I attended the Clinton Task Force "town meeting" at George Washington University, sponsored by the Robert Wood Johnson Foundation. Approximately 500 invited participants represented a spectrum of healthcare organizations. Notably, very few doctors were invited. The meeting was chaired by Vice President Gore. Three panels discussed every facet of healthcare. There was a strong antispecialist sentiment. A great deal of support was expressed for increasing the number and the role of family care physicians. This idea is epitomized by Dr. Steven Schroeder, President of the Robert Wood Johnson Foundation and host of the meeting, in an April 1, 1993 article in the *New England Journal of Medicine* entitled, "Specialty Distribution of U.S. Physicians: The Invisible Driver of Healthcare Costs." In keeping with the tone of the Clinton Task Force meeting, this article blamed much of America's rising healthcare costs on the 70 percent of American doctors who are specialists. This was at variance with a clear admonition by Dr. Alexander Walt, an invited panelist at the meeting and President of the American Board of Medical Specialties, that since World War II, specialists have been responsible for the great strength of American medicine. Specialists have created artificial knees and hips, PTCA, resection of aneurysms, bypass and laparoscopic surgery, all manner of imaging and a host of other therapeutic advances. Most people at that meeting, however, focused on the excesses of specialists rather than on the contributions that they have made. The journal, *Health Affairs*, published by Project Hope, recently released a 300-page supplement called, "Managed Competition: Healthcare Reform American Style," which I recommend if you really want to get a feeling for some of the ideas being considered by the Clinton Task Force. Much of the supplement is written by key members of the Clinton Task Force, such as Paul Starr and Walter Zelman, who favor competition under a budget, and by Alain Einthoven of Stanford. Einthoven is one of the principal architects of the concept of managed competition, which at this point is merely a theory and has never been tried. (Incidentally, Russell Baker recently wrote in the *New York Times* that managed competition is in itself a contradiction in terms. If competition is managed, it is by definition regulated and, therefore, not competition at all.)

There is an incisive article in the aforementioned issue of *Health Affairs* entitled, "An Iconoclastic View of Cost Containment," by

Joseph Newhouse, an economist and founding editor of *Health Economics*, who spent 25 years with the Rand Corporation. In his article, Newhouse debunks the widely held view that healthcare costs are increasing because of an aging population, wasteful administrative costs, the spread of health insurance and a surfeit of physicians. Nor does he believe that defensive medicine or expensive care of the terminally ill are major factors. Instead, he argues that medical costs are being driven up primarily by new technology. Newhouse thinks that managed competition without global budgets will not, except for a brief initial period, slow the rate of increased medical costs.

Victor Fuchs, a well-known health economist from Stanford, wrote an open letter to President Clinton that appeared in the April 1, 1993 issue of *JAMA*. Fuchs urged the President not to try to present a detailed health plan within 100 days. His letter was prophetic because a few days after it appeared, Mrs. Clinton announced that the May 1 deadline could not be met. A second deadline was not given. Fuchs warned that drug companies and physicians are not the main problems in the healthcare crisis. He cites three areas in which he believes change is needed. Fuchs wants healthcare disengaged from employment. Like Newhouse, he considers technological change the most important force behind increasing healthcare expenditures and that we need to develop institutional and scientific resources to define proper assessment and use of medical technologies. The third issue is that we need to learn to cope with an aging society. Fuchs questions whether market forces can create an equitable universal insurance system, harness technological change and cope with the potentially unlimited demand for healthcare by the elderly.

With this brief commentary, I do not pretend to give a comprehensive analysis of the problems facing healthcare reform. Rather, I cite these differing views to emphasize that healthcare reform at present is in a state of flux. No specific plan has yet been presented, nor do I believe that any plan exists in final form. But healthcare reform is needed and will occur. The Clinton administration is correct in recognizing this and in emphasizing it. It has, however, underestimated the complexity of the problem and the time required to find a solution. The Clinton approach, with its secret meetings and calculated exclusion of organized medicine from its deliberations, is unlikely to succeed. But the voice of medicine must be heard. I urge you all to become informed and to make your ideas known to your congressmen and senators. What medicine cannot afford is an attitude of resignation and futility. The American College of Cardiology and the American Medical Association must be active participants in the dynamic changes that are occurring in healthcare in the United States. But, the impact they will have — considering the present climate in Washington — is, at best, uncertain.

18

Medical Autonomy and Professionalism in Medicine: Can Their Decline Be Reversed?

December 1996

On the front page of the December 2, 1996 issue of *American Medical News*, there is a shocking article entitled, "Collective Bargaining: Managed Care Fuels Debate on Physician Unions." It describes a Tucson medical center with 142 staff doctors who will vote on forming a collective bargaining union to negotiate with their employer clinic and its owner, a California-based HMO. The article goes on to say that since the sale of their practice, "the doctors have been stripped of control over their hours and patient load and frozen out of medical decision-making." The labor relations board ruled that this loss of power showed that the staff doctors and their department chairman were truly employees and not supervisors and, therefore, they were authorized to vote to determine whether a union should be formed. One of the physicians who supported the union concept said that the union would attempt to reverse some of the managed care policies that were designed only to increase profits and not to improve patient care.

Current antitrust laws prevent independently practicing doctors from joining together to gain control of the financial and medical aspects of their practices. And yet a managed care organization or an insurance company can gain control of several hundred thousand "lives," as they put it, which is perhaps an accurate term since they do at times control life and death decisions for their insured. How is it that managed care organizations can decide which medical services can or cannot be rendered, even which doctor or hospital a patient can use, and yet practicing doctors are denied the right to resist collectively on behalf of their patients and denied the right to make purely medical decisions?

One of the Tucson doctors said that more and more physicians across the nation are coming to the same conclusion — that we need some sort of organization and structure that will allow us to act in concert against the total domination of managed care. In response to this point of view, an AMA trustee is quoted as saying that physicians are professionals and therefore should not delve into practices such as collective bargaining which could be construed as a union. I quite agree and I believe that many, if not most, physicians would concur that collective bargaining and the idea of a union are not in keeping with the kind of professionalism that we always believed medicine should represent. Unfortunately, the paradox of our times is that we are no longer being treated as professionals. Every facet of medical practice, both economic and professional, can be and is being dictated by the managed care industry. Our professionalism is being destroyed from without.

Ewe Reinhardt, a Princeton professor and healthcare economist, once said, "I do not think that most physicians recognize that the present system of competing health plans is the road to serfdom, particularly for specialists." His words were indeed prophetic. Doctors in other countries around the world have faced and are facing similar challenges and have perhaps reacted more realistically than we have in the United States. The British Medical Association, for example, negotiates professional and economic issues with the National Health Service and because of this activity, British physicians in the National Health Service are considered to be members of a union. But there are independently practicing doctors in Britain and many who spend part of their time in private practice even though they are members of the National Health Service. Recently, when a major American managed care company bought part ownership in a British insurance company, they sent a schedule to invasive and interventional cardiologists who practiced outside the National Health Service. The doctors merely said no to the schedule — something most American doctors have never done.

Medical professionalism is under siege throughout the world, but perhaps nowhere so much as it is in the United States. Thus far, there is no medical organization in this country that has been willing or able to make our Congress, our business leaders or the public aware of the devastating impact on medical care and, in the long run, on medical progress, that is imposed by the growing domination of mammoth managed care organizations and insurance companies. For them, the bottom line is the ultimate priority and the only priority.

This situation must be redressed, but to do so will require a change in Federal Trade Commission policies that will empower physicians to deal with managed care organizations and insurance companies on equal terms. The concept of a union has never been one that the medical profession has embraced or wants to embrace, but some vehicle is necessary to allow doctors to act in concert against the excesses of managed care. Perhaps no one said it better than Hamlet: "Diseases desperate grown by desperate appliance are relieved or not at all."

19

Ethics in Cardiovascular Medicine: The 29th American College of Cardiology Bethesda Conference

March 1998

In October 1997, the American College of Cardiology convened its 29th Bethesda Conference at Heart House, this one called, "Ethics in Cardiovascular Medicine." Bethesda Conferences are two-day colloquies on issues pertinent to cardiovascular medicine and surgery. The topic of the first conference in 1965 was "Standards of Physical Fitness of Air Crews" and subsequent conferences have included discussions of optimal electrocardiography, recommendations for determining eligibility for competitive athletes, cardiovascular abnormalities and cardiac transplantation. Bethesda Conference participants include some 60 fellows of the College and invited guests with expertise in the particular field being addressed.

The Bethesda Conference on ethics was chaired by Drs. William Parmley and Eugene Passamani. It was divided into three task forces. The first, which I had the privilege of co-chairing with Ward Kennedy, dealt with external influences on the practice of cardiology. The second, chaired by Spencer King and Dan Ullyot, considered the application of medical and surgical intervention near the end of life. And the third task force, chaired by Robert Roberts and Tom Ryan of Boston, focused on clinical research in a molecular era and the need to expand its ethical imperatives. There were plenary sessions for the entire group and each member was involved in one of the three task forces. The final results will be published in the *Journal of the American College of Cardiology*.

I would specifically like to discuss the group in which I participated, Task Force I that dealt with the external influences imposed by managed care on the practice of cardiology and cardiovascular surgery — a subject that I believe will be of great interest to both practicing and academic cardiologists. Managed care means different things to different people. In the context of this Bethesda Conference, the term managed care was used in its broadest sense to refer to a system of healthcare delivery, including both for-profit and non-profit managed care corporations and health insurance companies. Obviously, these various entities differ greatly in terms of the impact they have on the practice of cardiovascular medicine and surgery and on the manner in which they influence it.

Task Force I began by citing a 1997 *Journal of the American Medical Association* paper entitled, "Crisis, Ethics and the American Medical Association." Epitomizing the very reasons for this conference on ethics, this paper points out that American medicine is in crisis because the core values of the medical profession are being decided not by physicians, but by lawyers, judges and managed care administrators. The task force began its report with the statement: "Central to the relationship of the cardiologist to society is a covenant between doctor and patient." We unanimously agreed that the essence of this covenant was never stated better than it was by the late Cardinal Bernardin of Chicago when he spoke before the American Medical Association in December 1995, shortly before his death. The Cardinal said that the covenant between doctor and patient is grounded in the moral obligations that arise from the nature of the doctor-patient relationship and that these are moral obligations, as opposed to legal and contractual ones, because they are based on the fundamental human concept of right and wrong. Cardinal Bernardin acknowledged that it is not currently fashionable to think of medicine in terms of morality, yet morality is at the core of the doctor-patient relationship and the foundation of the medical profession. He asked this question: "Why do I insist on a moral model as opposed to the economic and contractual models now in vogue?" He answered with the salient elements that give the covenant between doctor and patient its moral status. Paramount among these is the reliance of the patient on the doctor. It is illness that compels the patient to put his or her fate in the hands of a doctor. The patient must rely not only on the technical competence of the doctor, but also on the doctor's moral compass and commitment to put the interests of the patient first. Cardinal Bernardin stated without equivocation that the doctor's personal commitment to the patient is based on a nontransferable fiduciary responsibility to protect the patient. He brought this precept down to the realities of today's medicine when he said, "Regardless of markets, government programs or network managers, patients depend on doctors for a personal commitment and for advocacy through an increasingly complex and impersonal system. In individual terms, the covenant between doctor and patient is the basis on which patients trust doctors. In social terms, the covenant is the ground for the public's continued respect and reliance on the profession of medicine."

Thus did Cardinal Bernardin's words prophetically set the stage for Task Force I to explore the external influences that affect this covenant between doctor and patient. One of these is the pressure placed on physicians by managed care to modify medical decisions. This can have an adverse effect on their patients, even including the denial of care. We also discussed how the various financial incentives to withhold or modify care may insidiously affect medical decisions, without even the physician's awareness.

Another fundamental issue considered by Task Force I was the relationship between the medical ethic and the business ethic. Capitalism, based on the theories of Adam Smith in the 18th century, has historically been motivated by profit in a free-market system. This principle dominates corporate philosophy as it seeks to achieve its goal of maximizing profit. But healthcare is unique to the business world because patients, now often called consumers, are highly vulnerable and easily exploited. A salient concept brought forth by the task force is that healthcare organizations must incorporate the ethical principles of beneficence and justice and protect patient rights even though profit may be their ultimate goal. The task force stated unequivocally that "the mutual acceptance of the principle that there must be no difference between the ethic of healthcare business and that of medicine would have a profound influence on the behavior of all those in the business of healthcare in any capacity." But the task force acknowledged that acceptance of these principles within the business healthcare community has not yet occurred or, if it has, it's in its infancy. Task Force I concluded that financial incentives have the potential to corrupt the moral values inherent in the physician-patient covenant and therefore, they must be disclosed.

The Bethesda Conference strongly supports the principles expressed in the November 1997 Presidents Advisory Commission on Protection and Quality in the Healthcare Industry. The several categories of rights and responsibilities expressed in this document are outlined in the Bethesda Conference Report, although the conference recognizes that legislation alone cannot replace a universal code of ethics for the healthcare industry. Task Force I challenged doctors to articulate medicine's ethical code and challenged managed care organizations to move toward greater and more enlightened social responsibility. To this end, the conference accepted eight recommendations by Task Force I, all of which were approved in a plenary session by a vote of more than 70 percent of all those participating in the conference.

Briefly stated, the recommendation are as follows: Establish a national dialogue on ethical standards to be followed throughout the healthcare industry and specifically by all those involved directly or indirectly in patient care; redirect financial incentives from withholding care to improving care; require full disclosure of the mechanism of distribution and the actual dollar amounts of financial incentives and disincentives offered to physicians; require an independent expeditor for the appeal process to resolve patient disputes; protect physicians against sanctions when they appeal medical decisions on behalf of their patients; require full disclosure of medical services that are covered; and finally, confirm the patient's right of direct access to reasonable specialty care.

The Bethesda Conference has set forth ethical standards and goals, many of which are still being violated in a medical environment radically different from the one that existed only a decade or two ago. An approach toward achieving these goals has been enunciated. However, I must say reluctantly that only the most unrestrained optimist can really believe that these ethical goals and standards can be achieved in the foreseeable future. Nevertheless, I urge you to read the report of the 29th Bethesda Conference, to embrace the principles for which it stands and to work to implement them — no matter how long it takes or how difficult these tasks may be.

20

The AMA and the U.S. Congress: Responding to the Tyranny of the HMO-Insurance Complex

June 1999

On June 23, 1999, an action taken by the American Medical Association House of Delegates in Chicago became front-page and prime-time news throughout the country. The AMA had embraced the principle of a union for doctors. And while the AMA House of Delegates was endorsing this principle of collective bargaining for doctors, the Congress of the United States was engaged in rancorous and partisan debate over the issue of a bill of rights for patients. Both of these deliberative bodies were responding to the growing domination and control of healthcare in the United States by the managed care-insurance complex.

Representing an organization of some 290,000 doctors, the AMA House of Delegates abandoned its long-standing position against unions for doctors, recognizing that in the present climate, doctors simply cannot cope with the power — or perhaps I should have said, the tyranny — of managed care. In his June 22, 1999 statement before the Judiciary Committee of the U.S. House of Representatives, Dr. Radcliffe Anderson, Executive Vice President of the AMA, said that in many cities in the United States, doctors are confronted by healthcare plans so dominant that they refuse to negotiate any contract terms, even those addressing vitally important patient care issues. Doctors are simply being given "take it or leave it" contracts to which no one in any other business situation would agree. Dr. Anderson went on to say that the power of health plans to unilaterally determine the kind of healthcare patients will receive in the United States is virtually absolute. He illustrated this point by citing the proposed Prudential HealthCare acquisition by Aetna U.S. Healthcare, which would create a plan covering one in ten privately insured persons in the United States. In Houston, Aetna-Prudential would control over 50 percent of the market with 66 percent of fully funded commercial HMO patients, the closest competitor being United Health

Care with a 9 percent market share. In addition, Aetna-Prudential would have between 30 and 59 percent of the HMO markets in Atlanta, Orlando and in several counties in New Jersey.

Mindful of this, federal approval of the Aetna U.S. Healthcare $1 billion purchase of Prudential HealthCare has been given only after an agreement by the new combined company to divest its plans in Dallas and Houston. Even before the Aetna-Prudential merger, the five largest insurers had more than 50 percent of the market in 23 states and more than 70 percent in 16 states. Ewe Reinhardt, the well-known but mercurial and unpredictable Princeton economist who is not always friendly to medicine, said that the Aetna-Prudential merger would control one-third of the New York healthcare market, effectively eliminating any real competition.

Dr. Anderson told the House of Representatives that by the year 2002, there will be 101 million HMO enrollees, up from 81 million in 1997, and that the Preferred Provider Organization (PPO) enrollment at the end of 1996 was 98 million. He added that there are simply not enough patients outside managed care to provide most physicians with enough patient volume to survive in practice. It is in this milieu that the AMA has endorsed the principle of collective bargaining for doctors — even though at present, this principle applies only to employed doctors such as hospital residents and those working at HMOs. Doctors in private practice cannot bargain collectively under present Federal Trade Commission regulations. Doctors who attempt it or even get together to plan a common strategy face the threat of criminal prosecution.

In spite of the media's frequent use of the words "union" and "unionization," the AMA does not advocate, nor has it voted for, a traditional labor union. Furthermore, the AMA has forsworn the right to strike, the traditional weapon of labor unions, because it refuses to compromise or neglect patient care during the negotiating process. But the AMA will forthwith begin to create an organization to carry out collective bargaining by employed physicians.

Employed doctors have had the right to form collective bargaining units even before the AMA's current action. The real challenge will be to pass legislation that changes the rules under which the Federal Trade Commission operates because only then will practicing doctors have the right to bargain collectively. The instrument for removing these restrictions is House Bill 1304, introduced by Congressmen Tom Campbell (R-CA) and John Conyers (D-MI). Bill 1304 has broad bipartisan co-sponsorship and support and is aptly titled, "The Quality Healthcare Coalition Act of 1999." Campbell and Conyers have said, "This legislation is the best way to let market forces deal with the complaints so many healthcare professionals have against the HMOs." House Bill 1304 is strongly supported by the AMA, by the American College of Cardiology and by many other major medical organizations. It will enable practicing doctors to negotiate contracts with health plans and hospitals without violating antitrust laws. It should not be forgotten that HMOs and health insurers already have antitrust protections under the McCarren-Ferguson Act. House Bill 1304 would merely give practicing doctors this same protection.

In spite of the compelling arguments presented in favor of Bill 1304 by Drs. Anderson and Smoak, the American Bar Association appeared before the House Judiciary Committee, expressing its vigorous opposition. The American Bar Association said that the present antitrust law is essential in preserving the competitive process that will assure that healthcare markets respond, as they put it, in a dynamic and efficient way to consumer preferences.

At the June 22nd hearing of the House Committee on the Campbell-Conyers Bill, the Chairman of the Federal Trade Commission called it "an unprecedented departure from economic policy and a disproportionate response to the problem." President Clinton's own Department of Justice argued that the bill will result in price-fixing and boycotting. All of this dramatically shows how difficult the battle will be to pass House Bill 1304 over the opposition of the Federal Trade Commission, the U.S. Department of Justice, the American Bar Association and the powerful managed care-insurance complex lobby.

I find it hypocritical of the Department of Justice to take the position that the Campbell-Conyers Bill will result in price-fixing. The reality is that the practice of medicine is perhaps the only part of our otherwise free enterprise system where there is already price-fixing, both by government and private sectors. Rather than fixing prices, the repeal of Federal Trade Commission restrictions on doctor collective bargaining would enable physicians to resist the already draconian price-fixing imposed both by government and the HMO-insurance complex.

The Campbell-Conyers Bill is not the only legislation before the Congress of vital importance to the healthcare industry. There is the "Patients' Bill of Rights," around which swirls a highly charged and partisan struggle wherein Democrats and Republicans alike appear to respond more to the desires of special interests than to the needs of patients.

I cannot let this moment pass without saying that the most important element in the Patients' Bill of Rights is to make the HMO-insurance complex accountable for its decisions that affect patient care, just as doctors are accountable. And the only way for this accountability to have a real impact is for patients to have the right to sue when vital healthcare is delayed or denied. Nothing will influence the performance of the HMO-insurance complex as much as accountability — accountability that can be enforced only by a court of law.

For those who think that the American Medical Association and American medicine in general are alone in their struggle for an environment more favorable to optimal patient care or that the British healthcare system is entirely different from our own, an article in the London *Times* on July 6, 1999 may give some comfort. At its annual meeting in Belfast, the British Medical Association (BMA) gave a standing ovation to their President, Ian Bogle, when he accused Prime Minister Tony Blair of introducing policies without consultation that perpetuate bureaucracy and force doctors to work at a pace that is contrary to safe medical practice. We've heard similar complaints in the United States. Dr. Bogle said that the government had introduced "an iniquitous internal market, a General Practitioner contract underpinned by meaningless targets and unnecessary bureaucracy in a management-driven system that shifted the focus of our jobs away from patient care toward administration." This echoes the refrain heard in the United States. At the meeting of the BMA, 550 delegates voted unanimously to condemn the government for its practices in dealing with the British healthcare system.

If there is a common thread through all of the issues that I've discussed, it is the need for balance between the overwhelming power of government and the HMO insurance complex and the presently powerless medical and patient communities. To achieve this goal, three things are necessary. First, the Federal Trade Commission policies must be changed to allow physicians and other healthcare professionals to bargain collectively. Second, there must be relief from the present system that gives both government and the private sector limitless unilateral ability to fix prices throughout the healthcare industry without recourse by doctors. Third, a Patients' Bill of Rights must be passed that includes accountability of the managed care-insurance complex — and accountability before a court of law. Nothing short of acceptance of these three principles can redress the current inequities in the American healthcare system.

History teaches that tyranny and injustice inevitably lead to revolution. Within the short span of two weeks in the summer of 1999, both the American Medical Association and the British Medical Association have, at long last, begun this revolution. In so doing, they deserve not only our applause but our vigorous support. This support can best be expressed by personal contact with our representatives in Congress and with our patients. After all — it is up to us.

21

Managing the Excesses of Managed Care: The Courts or the Congress?

September 1999

In the previous editorial, I discussed the acrimonious and partisan debate in Congress over what some are calling a "Patients' Bill of Rights." While both political parties seem to agree that patients and doctors need protection from the growing power of the managed care-insurance complex, there is little consensus on the nature and degree of this protection. One of the most contentious elements of the debate before the Congress is the accountability of managed care organizations when harm or death occurs to patients whose care, specifically recommended by doctors, was delayed or denied. While the "right to sue" may be the most visible flash point in the congressional debate, a more fundamental issue may be what role the courts should play in defining and perhaps limiting the power of the managed care-insurance complex. Also, it is necessary to determine the extent to which the managed care industry should be permitted to control medical decisions and, in essence, control the practice of medicine and the very nature of healthcare in the United States.

Exploring this complex issue, there is a thoughtful, comprehensive and incisive paper by Peter Jacobson of the University of Michigan School of Public Health, published in the July/August, 1999 issue of *Health Affairs* entitled, "Legal Challenges to Managed Care Cost-Containment Programs — An Initial Assessment: Are the Courts Willing to Hold Health Plans Accountable for Delay and Denial of Care." Jacobson sets the stage in the prologue to his article: "In a legal system as freewheeling as America's, the protection afforded health plans under the Employee Retirement Income Security Act (ERISA) is viewed by many as anomalous. Under this provision, health plans covering approximately 140 million Americans are largely protected from liability in lawsuits involving denial of medically necessary care." This issue prompted Senate Minority Leader Tom Daschle to ask, "Why is it that we only give immunity to diplomats and HMOs?" Based on his study, Jacobson suggests that to date, the courts have not systematically impeded managed care programs. Rather the courts have tended to defer to market forces, however unbalanced they may be.

Jacobson's paper addresses three questions. How have the courts responded thus far to legal challenges by patients to cost-containment programs? What are the emerging issues in litigation between doctors and managed care? What are the policy implications of such litigation? To answer these questions, Jacobson reviewed judicial decisions in healthcare cases that challenged managed care cost-containment programs using Westlaw and Lexis-Nexis data to study 500 from a total universe of 3800 potential cases According to the data presented, it seems very likely that the courts will become more and more deeply involved in healthcare issues as managed care expands. Jacobson points out, I think very wisely, that in the current managed care environment, a conflict is occurring between population-based cost-containment and healthcare services for individuals. Both patients and doctors are stakeholders whose interests will inevitably be brought before courts of law. There will be conflicts over both resource allocation and physician autonomy. In addition, the backlash against managed care is generating legislation and regulation to protect patients' rights that the courts will eventually have to interpret.

How the courts should respond to challenges to cost-containment initiatives by managed care has been the subject of intense scholarly debate. Some analysts consider that the courts have sided with insurers in deciding whether or not contested benefits should be covered. Jacobson also concludes from his research that the courts have been more deferential to managed care than to plaintiffs, whether they are patients or doctors.

One of the pivotal issues before the courts is the question of the ERISA preemption. ERISA governs private employer-sponsored benefit plans, including health plans offered by self-insured firms that cover more than 65 percent of the insured population. But ERISA was never really intended to apply to healthcare. Rather, it was designed to protect employee pension plans. Nevertheless, as ERISA is now interpreted, it preempts state laws including personal injury claims that relate to employer benefit plans — a very broad interpretation indeed. Jacobson believes that the ERISA preemption creates a regulatory vacuum in which states cannot act and for which there is no federal regulatory presence governing individual litigation against HMOs. More recently, the courts have ruled that challenges to the technical quality of healthcare do not involve the administration of benefits plans and therefore cannot be preempted, thus allowing access to the state courts. For example, discharging a patient early may be construed as a clinical decision instead of a benefits decision and therefore amenable to state court jurisdiction.

Further challenges exist on the issue of financial incentives. The question is whether a patient can sue a physician or healthcare plan for negligence based on financially motivated clinical decisions. Up to this point, however, in no case has liability actually been determined based on financial motivation. To illustrate this, Jacobson cites a case against the Kaiser Foundation Health Plan of the Mid-Atlantic States in which a patient challenged a Kaiser Foundation incentive program that encouraged physicians not to prescribe certain expensive tests or to refer patients to specialists. The court found that even though the claim was valid, because it was protected by the ERISA shield, the plaintiff was denied.

The question of utilization management imposed by managed care has also been tested in court. In general, the courts have ruled that the utilization management is a benefit, a financial matter rather than a clinical decision. This approach tends to give health plans wide latitude to control costs, as Jacobson puts it, at the expense of both the patient's access to care and the treating physician's clinical autonomy.

There is the further legal issue of physicians versus managed care organizations. In this arena, doctors have tried to invoke antitrust doctrines to protect against measures such as selective contracting and economic credentialing. But the courts have held that these actions are allowable, thereby placing cost-containment objectives above the interests of physicians. In bioethics cases, the courts have, at times, been willing to make decisions that many thought should be left to the legislative bodies. On the other hand, in some ERISA cases, judges have complained vigorously that the ERISA preemption unjustly prevents courts from holding managed care accountable, and yet they have largely deferred to Congress to change the ERISA preemption rather than to use their own judicial powers.

Jacobson's extensive and detailed review of some 500 cases concludes that managed care accountability resides primarily with the Congress and state legislatures and not with the courts. This leads to a rather ironic change in the attitude of physicians. Doctors who have in the past resented medical liability doctrine as interpreted by the courts now turn to the courts as their best hope for restraining managed care and thus retaining their autonomy in medical practice.

Jacobson believes that the legislative process offers a far greater probability of limiting HMO power than can be expected from the courts in the foreseeable future. If this indeed is true, there is at least one hopeful prospect, and that is the burgeoning bipartisan movement in the Congress to do what the courts have as yet been unwilling to do — to defend patient and doctor prerogatives against the now pervasive power of managed care. Only time will tell whether these bipartisan efforts can survive the powerful HMO-insurance complex lobby.

22

An American Obsession: Minimize Hospitalization and Length of Stay

September 1996

octors in all fields — and perhaps especially those in cardiology and cardiovascular surgery who have practiced for several years now — are under pressure from what might be called the cost-containment police. Most doctors would undoubtedly agree that the two most strident and often-repeated injunctions of cost containment are to keep patients out of the hospital and, if they are admitted, get them out as quickly as possible. In fact, the most highly prized statistic for cardiac surgical programs is a short length of stay, second only to a low mortality rate.

This virtually unchallenged approach to medical cost reduction is confronted in an article in the Summer 1996 edition of *Health Affairs*, written by the well-known health economist and Professor of Political Economy at Princeton, Uwe Reinhardt. Reinhardt presents his ideas under the provocative title, "Spending More Through 'Cost Control': Our Obsessive Quest to Gut the Hospital." He mentions that a year ago, when he was at an international conference on American medical cost-control techniques, a European doctor — whose country spends about 9 percent of its Gross National Product (GNP) on healthcare today, the same as it did in 1980 — asked what percentage of the GNP the United States spent on healthcare 10 years ago and what it spends today. When told that in 1980 we spent 9 percent and now we spend about 14 percent, the European doctor, with a barely concealed smirk, responded, "Tell me more about your wondrous cost-control techniques, please tell me more!" As an example of these "wondrous" cost-control techniques, Reinhardt mentions the California experience, generally considered to be a most progressive method of controlling medical costs through the aggressive use of managed care techniques. Reinhardt points out that a recent Lewin-VHI study found that so far, all of California's efforts have merely reduced its average per capita healthcare spending to the national level.

Among employee benefit managers of large corporations, insurance companies and managed care programs and even among hospital executives, it is axiomatic that effective cost control depends on two easily understood economic benchmarks — total hospital admissions per thousand and average length of stay per hospital episode. Reinhardt adds that any strategy that achieves the lowest rate of inpatient days per capita is immediately labeled the best practice. Between 1980 and 1995, this approach reduced inpatient admissions per thousand and the average length of stay by 20 percent each. As a result, inpatient days per thousand in the United States have declined by 40 percent, according to the American Hospital Association. It is this obsession, to use Reinhardt's word, that has led many managed care organizations to mandate a 24-hour hospital stay for a normal birth and 48 hours for a cesarean section, despite objections from both mothers and doctors. It is this obsession that led New Jersey Governor Christine Todd Whitman, after signing a law preventing such practices, to say that she was merely imposing a measure of common sense on the private sector. More recently, the United States Congress passed similar legislation.

Nations with a much lower level of healthcare spending have far more hospital beds, more hospital admissions and more inhospital days per capita than does the United States. While Reinhardt concedes that this in itself doesn't prove anything, it does suggest that the emphasis on hospital admissions and length of stay may not be the total answer to effective cost containment. He offers an interesting hypothesis and one that is contrary to the conventional wisdom of cost control through limited hospital admissions and length of stay. Reinhardt contests the oft-repeated statement that hospitals are very expensive places. Rather, he believes that they are very expensive at certain times and relatively inexpensive at others, depending on what is happening to the patient. He believes that flat per diem rates, negotiated by hospitals, insurance companies and managed care organizations, do not reflect the actual profile of a cost per day during the entire hospital stay. A flat rate of, say, $1000 to $1500 a day is structured to cover the incremental cost per hospital day and also to recover the hospital's fixed overhead. By the incremental cost of a unit of output — an economic term for an inpatient day — Reinhardt means the cost that would be avoided if that particular hospital day were not added. For example, for the second or third day of a maternity stay, the incremental cost would most likely not exceed $200 a day. Fixed overhead, on the other hand, is a cost that does not change with the number of hospital days. In other words, fixed overhead continues whether the bed is occupied or not. As Reinhardt points out, the incremental cost per inpatient day during the convalescent phase is relatively low, therefore, the flat per diem rate is what he calls a perverse form of pricing.

Never lacking in the ability or desire to turn a phrase, Reinhardt says that in the end, the high flat negotiated per diem charge, which may be $1000 to $1500 a day for this discretionary or incremental day, will drive even church-going HMO executives to kick new mothers and their babies out of the hospital. If charges for the discretionary day were realistic, as Reinhardt believes they should be, there would be less pressure to shorten hospital stay and the consequences of doing so would not occur.

Reinhardt observes that two industries have arisen as a result of the pressures to minimize hospital stay — home healthcare and subacute care industries. He asks the reader to imagine how a budding health-care entrepreneur planning a home healthcare service, for example, might react when he realizes that all he has to do to compete with hos-pitals is charge less than their $1000 a day rate. Even at a cost of as much as $400 a day, he could most likely turn a handsome profit, even if convalescent patients had to be washed and fed intravenously in their homes, and even if the patients required rather extensive health serv-ices. Compared with a $1000 hospital day, this new service would be in great demand — and indeed it is.

Reinhardt believes this kind of reasoning is possible because the hospital charge for the late incremental day is unrealistically inflated. He makes the point that since 1980, during which time there has been a 40 percent reduction in inhospital days per thousand population, U.S. spending has still gone from 9 percent of the GNP to the current 14 percent in spite of this drastic reduction in per capita hospitalization and length of stay. He contends that healthcare spending has risen, not necessarily in spite of reduction of hospital inpatient care, but at least in part because of it. He reminds us that while Medicare uses fixed di-agnostic related groups (DRGs) for inpatient reimbursement for home and subacute care, it still pays a full cost plus. And it is this surrender of the key to the public treasury, as Reinhardt puts it, that has made subacute and home healthcare the fastest-growing components of the Medicare program. I might add that this sector is the least monitored and controlled of today's programs and perhaps the most abused. The DRG program has given hospitals an incentive to discharge patients as soon as possible into either subacute care or home care and that incen-tive, according to Reinhardt, is even stronger when the hospital pro-vides all three components — inpatient, subacute and home care. While the hospital may be constrained by DRGs on its inpatient charges, in a sense it has a blank check because the subacute and home care is assumed, no matter what, to be less expensive than inpatient hospital care.

In summary, Reinhardt's thesis is that the home healthcare and subacute care industries would not have grown as rapidly as they did and probably would not have become nearly so profitable had it not been for the pressures to reduce length of hospital stay, driven by fallacious flat per diem billing practices — in other words, not billing realistically for the relatively low incremental cost of late hospital days. In my judgment, none of this should be construed as a denial that many unnecessary hospitalizations have justifiably been eliminated and excessive length of stays modified. But Reinhardt's views are refreshing to many of us who have long been aware of the unseemly practice of same-day admission for elderly and frail open heart patients and dismissing patients before doctors think they're medically ready, causing them to be relegated to inconvenient, often inadequate and exorbitantly priced home and subacute care facilities. While patients may survive these practices, they are often subjected to great distress and discomfort.

Though many of us may have sensed intuitively what Reinhardt has stated in economic terms, and even though other economists may disagree with what he has said, his strongly worded argument may trigger a reappraisal of some practices in healthcare reform that have been accepted far too readily. In the final analysis, as Reinhardt suggests, these practices may be hard on patients without even saving as much money as has been assumed.

23

Three-Day Post-MI Hospital Stay: How Safe? Which Patient? Who Decides and on What Evidence?

March 2000

In the March 16, 2000 issue of the New England Journal of Medicine, there is an article entitled, "Cost Effectiveness of Early Discharge After Uncomplicated Acute Myocardial Infarction," written by Kristin Newby and her associates from Duke Clinical Research Institute in Durham, North Carolina. The article's premise is that reducing the length of hospitalization in acute myocardial infarction (MI) can reduce long-term costs, but there are insufficient data to prove that reduction of length of stay can occur without compromising patient outcomes. The authors, quite correctly I believe, point out that despite this lack of evidence, healthcare providers are developing cost-cutting guidelines to shorten hospital stays after acute MI. (By providers, I presume the authors mean third-party payers, hospitals and doctors.) It is pressure from third-party payers, however, that causes hospitals to pressure doctors to shorten hospital stays. Doctors in turn are seeking evidence as to how short the post-MI stay can be without adversely affecting the patient's ultimate outcome and how to identify those patients for whom the three-day stay is safe.

Using Gusto I data, the authors found some 22,000 patients who had an uncomplicated course for 72 hours after thrombolysis. They then applied a decision-analytic model to determine the cost-effectiveness of an additional day of hospitalization in this group. They defined the benefit of an additional day — that is, a fourth day in the hospital — on the basis of inhospital resuscitation between 72 and 96 hours after cardiac arrest. Lifetime survival was estimated from one-year Gusto I survival data. Sixteen patients among the more than 22,000 in the cohort had major ventricular arrhythmias, 13 of whom were successfully resuscitated. The presumption was that the only discernible benefit of hospitalizing some 22,000 patients for a fourth day was to those 13 patients who were successfully resuscitated from cardiac arrest.

For this 22,000-patient cohort, the authors' projections indicate that this represents only a 0.006 year of life saved at a cost of $624 per day, or slightly more than $105,000 per year of life saved. The authors consider this cost-ineffective and concluded, therefore, that a fourth day of hospitalization would be "economically attractive only if the costs could be reduced by more than 50 percent, or if a high-risk subgroup could be identified in which case estimated survival benefit would be doubled." They go on to say that this $105,000 per year of life saved is economically unattractive compared with other strategies for managing acute myocardial infarction. For example, the use of altepase instead of streptokinase results in a cost of $33,000 per year of life saved, and the use of angioplasty for acute MI in middle-aged men carries a cost of $52,000 per year of life saved.

The authors point out quite correctly that a cost-effective analysis of this kind requires that several assumptions be made. The validity of these assumptions is critical to the validity of results. They list seven such assumptions, some of which deserve special mention. The first assumption is that among patients with an uncomplicated 72-hour course, the rate of cardiac events, including cardiac arrest in the hospital, would be the same for those patients dismissed after 72 hours. Another assumption is that the primary benefit of hospitalization beyond 72 hours is prompt resuscitation if cardiac arrest occurs. It is further assumed that after discharge, patients who had reinfarction, stroke or recurrent ischemia, heart failure or complications other than cardiac arrest, could be hospitalized promptly enough so that any change in long-term outcome or costs would not occur. I might add that in the absence of data on the course of these patients following three-day dismissal, this assumption requires, if not a leap of faith, at least a considerable amount of optimism.

In reviewing their assumptions, the authors concede that in a three-day stay, risk stratification, teaching and rehabilitation would be carried out with substantial difficulty in many centers. Their model assumes, however, that in the long run, hospitals would be able to incorporate all these activities in a three-day period without a major increase in cost. They warn that long-term follow-up of these early-discharge patients is essential to assure that short-term gains and reduced costs do not occur at the expense of long-term clinical outcomes. This is especially important because the three-day length of stay is based on a complicated series of projections and assumptions rather than on hard evidence.

Unfortunately, this uncertainty about the safety of the three-day length of stay is not the message that comes through to the public and perhaps even more importantly, to the insurers and HMOs who watch very carefully for any signal that might suggest an opportunity to reduce length of stay. For example, in the *Wall Street Journal* of March 16,

2000, the headline on the article that was reporting this paper read, "Some heart attack patients found able to be released after just three days." The article was quite perceptive in recalling that three years ago, following a cost-effectiveness study, insurers began pressuring hospitals for a 24-hour postpartum release, which ultimately led to a national uproar and congressional legislation that extended the maternity stay.

In the *New England Journal of Medicine* for March 16, 2000, there is an editorial critique of the Newby paper by Elliott Antman of The Brigham and Women's Hospital and Karen Kuntz of the Harvard School of Public Health in which the authors give some historical perspective on the progress that has been made since the 1950s in reducing length of stay after acute MI. They recall the doctrine prevalent at that time that an infarcted heart, like a fractured bone, was best treated by immobilization. This meant a four- to six-week hospital stay at bedrest with all the associated complications, including embolism and debility. But that was a different era with different alternatives for treatment. Perhaps not many will recall the furor caused by the publication of a *JAMA* article written by the legendary Dr. Sam Levine and his then-young associate Bernie Lown, that called for "armchair treatment" of acute coronary thrombosis. At the time, this was a major, albeit extremely controversial, advance in which an armchair was placed next to the hospital bed and the patient lifted into it to assume a more comfortable seated posture. The duration of stay was gradually reduced over the years to five or six days and then to the three-day period under discussion.

As the Antman-Kuntz editorial suggests, the length of the post-MI stay issue has political, ethical and legal implications and is of critical importance in allocating resources — and I might add, is of special interest to insurers and to their profitability. The editorial states categorically, and I believe very wisely, that this cost-effective analysis must be viewed as a guide rather than as a mandate for practice. The editorial also raises some important questions about the proposed three-day stay that might limit clinicians in adjusting the dose of beta blockers, ACE inhibitors, and other medications that are critically important in long-term management. In considering the wide range of implications of the Newby study, it is of paramount importance that the care of the myocardial infarction patient not be reduced to an assembly-line approach that focuses only on whether or not a cardiac arrest occurs on the fourth day and implies that the only benefit of an extra day or two of hospitalization is the treatment of cardiac arrest.

A myocardial infarction, however uncomplicated, has a tremendous impact on both the patient and family. In the public mind, and in reality, a heart attack is a brush with death and a permanent reminder of one's mortality. It takes time for a patient to come to terms with such an event that is a watershed experience in life — even if it has a relatively benign course and a lack of complications. Helping a patient understand what a heart attack is, how to adjust to it, and to instill some optimism about the future, may be as important as some of the medicines that are prescribed. This is a difficult task to achieve in three days. Anyone who has worked in a coronary care unit knows that patients usually remember very little of what is said to them during those first three days. Beyond that, not every patient has a home situation that can make a three-day dismissal possible. That a patient simply may not be psychologically ready for dismissal in three days is also important, although this is difficult to measure and probably of little interest to the third-party payer. It should, however, be of great interest to the doctor as the patient's advocate.

The Newby paper is quite emphatic that the conclusions presented apply only to a specific group of patients who meet the Gusto I inclusion criteria and who have undergone thrombolysis and an uncomplicated three-day course. These results cannot be generalized to other patients with acute MI.

Returning to the authors' statement that the $105,000 per year of life saved does not meet conventional standards and does not conform to the "economically attractive threshold of less than $50,000 a year per life saved," I submit that society has really never established such a threshold. The authors themselves remind us that the use of smoke detectors in homes is estimated to cost some $240,000 a year per life saved. In the same vein, the Antman-Kuntz editorial notes that society is apparently willing to spend more for toxin control than for some medical interventions, as shown by the $834,000 per year of life saved, which is what it costs to control emissions from radionucleides, according to the Department of Energy. And the American Cancer Society's recommendation of annual mammography for women beginning at age 40, rather than 50, would cost more than $150,000 a year for each life saved.

The Newby paper and the Antman-Kuntz commentaries are important in helping to define minimal but safe duration of hospitalization after heart attack. Both highlight the need for further research and for getting hard data in this area. But at this time, there is no incontrovertible evidence upon which to impose arbitrary hospital discharge policy for the patient who has experienced acute myocardial infarction, however uncomplicated. Perhaps it should not be forgotten that it is the doctor at the bedside who knows about this patient and therefore, may have a better sense of whether a specific patient needs a day or two more in the hospital than can be gleaned from data sheets based on thousands of cases.

24

On the Continuing Cholesterol Controversy

November 1989

I received a letter from Dr. Bruce Wilson, Assistant Professor and Director of the University of Pittsburgh Heart Institute and an avid ACCEL listener, in which he wrote, "The cholesterol controversy has been a recurrent theme on your programs and I'm glad to hear that it remains, at least from your perspective, a controversy." Dr. Wilson also sent me an article called, "The Cholesterol Myth," by Thomas J. Moore. This article, the cover story in this past September's *Atlantic Monthly*, is a preview of a chapter in Moore's upcoming book, *Heart Failure*, to be published by Random House. The book is controversial not only with regard to cholesterol, but because it deals with many behind the scene intrigues both inside and outside of medicine's ivory towers.

Moore's iconoclastic views are epitomized by the message on *Atlantic's* cover: "Lowering your cholesterol is next to impossible with diet, and often dangerous with drugs — and it won't make you live any longer." Moore contends that the value of lowering cholesterol in the general population has been vastly overstated. He claims that many millions of people may be receiving drugs they don't really need that have potentially harmful and as yet undefined side effects. Whether or not there is any merit in what Moore is saying, he has vaulted the cholesterol controversy into the public limelight. Dr. Claude Lefant, Director of the National Heart, Lung and Blood Institute, takes sharp issue with Moore. "This article," he says, "includes a series of errors and omissions about the National Heart, Lung, and Blood Institute, about the National Cholesterol Education Program, and about the science which supports that program."

The debate also rages in the public press. The *New York Times* ran an editorial on September 14, 1989 entitled, "Doubts about the Cholesterol Crusade." Later that month, the *Times* headlined an article, "Who Should Lower Cholesterol?" On October 9, 1989, the cover story in *Business Week* asked, "Can Corn Flakes Cure Cancer?" The subtitle answered, "Of course not, but health claims purported to reduce cholesterol are becoming ridiculous." About the same time, *Newsweek* featured an article entitled, "Cholesterol Confusion," and asked the question, "Are our efforts to prevent heart disease through diet and drugs a waste of time?"

These challenges to what might be called conventional cholesterol wisdom are not limited to the media. In the September 1989 issue of the *Archives of Internal Medicine*, there is an article by Drs. David Malenka and John Baron from Dartmouth, entitled, "Cholesterol and Coronary Heart Disease: Attributable Risk of Diet and Drugs." In it, they note that the efficacy of treating hypercholesterolemia is often expressed in relative terms, such as the ratio of risk in treated versus untreated populations. However, the clinical impact of treatment is best measured by the differences in risk, known as the attributable risk reduction. They cite an example: "The doctor may note that treatment of hypercholesterolemia can reduce the risk of coronary disease by 50 percent. The use of such relative measures is a carryover from classical epidemiology where relative risk is useful in measuring the strength of an association between disease and exposure. However, the relative risk is not a clinically relevant measure of effectiveness."

On September 7, 1989, the *New England Journal of Medicine* printed an article entitled, "Treating Hypercholesterolemia: How Should Practicing Physicians Interpret the Published Data?" The author, Dr. Allan Brett of New England Deaconess Hospital in Boston, believes that it's very important for clinicians to examine how published results are expressed, what is emphasized and what is left unsaid. Dr. Brett gives two examples pertinent to the cholesterol problem. The first is the famous 1984 Lipid Research Clinics (LRC) trial where a 1.7 percent absolute difference in endpoints was described as a 19 percent reduction. In the Helsinki Gemfibrozil trial, a 1.4 percent absolute difference, derived from a drop in coronary events from 4.1 percent in the placebo group to 2.7 percent in the Gemfibrozil group, was expressed as a 34 percent drop in coronary events. Brett notes that while this language is technically accurate, it may operate subliminally to magnify the effect of the intervention. The difference in outcomes may be statistically significant, but emphasizing a relative reduction focuses attention exclusively on the small proportion of patients who had a morbid event. Pharmaceutical advertising also often highlights relative risk reductions. As an example, Brett refers to the widely circulated advertisement for cholestyramine that cites the LRC trial and proclaims that the drug reduces coronary disease up to 39 percent. Again, relative risk is emphasized and this time, for a very small subgroup of the study. Brett points out that many people must be treated to benefit a relatively few and he questions the value of treating a large population to benefit only 1 or 2 percent.

The *Annals of Internal Medicine* for October 15, 1989 featured an editorial by Dr. Alan Garber of Stanford, entitled, "Where to Draw the Line Against Cholesterol?" Gerber refers to a recent report that was issued by the Toronto Working Group on cholesterol in the management of asymptomatic hypercholesteremia advocating a more selective approach to testing and treating hypercholesterolemia than our National Cholesterol Education Program does. Dr. Garber asks several very important questions: Can we infer that controlling hypercholesterolemia will prevent coronary disease in women, young men and elderly men? Do we need more direct evidence before we can recommend screening and treatment of population groups who have not as yet been studied in randomized trials? What will it cost to implement an aggressive approach? To all three questions, Dr. Garber answers, "the experts disagree."

These articles from the medical literature and those I have quoted from the lay press seem to challenge the almost evangelical approach to reducing cholesterol levels of the entire population. They question the concept of using relative risk reduction as a basis for making clinical decisions in individual patients.

25

The Imperative for Lipid Lowering in the Treatment of Coronary Artery Disease

June 1995

"Lower Patients' Cholesterol Now. Trial Evidence Shows Clear Benefits from Secondary Prevention." This is the title of the lead editorial in the *British Medical Journal* on May 20, 1995 — an editorial that reinforces a position now widely held throughout the cardiology community. While there is broad consensus for lipid lowering for secondary prevention, in reality, secondary prevention is a euphemism for treatment of patients with established coronary disease.

The *BMJ* editorial begins by stating that the lipid hypothesis — namely, that elevated plasma cholesterol levels are associated with a high incidence of atherosclerosis and risk of coronary disease — is no longer in question. The editorial sets forth in unequivocal language that the results of several 1994 tests remove from the controversial category a clearly defined segment of patients — those with established coronary heart disease. Among these studies, the flagship trial is the Scandinavian Simvastatin Survival Study (known as the 4S study), in which some 4400 patients with coronary disease and cholesterol levels that ranged from 5.5 to 8.0 millimols (or in American parlance, approximately 220 to 320 milligrams percent) had a substantial reduction, not only in mortality, but also in cardiovascular events, and there was no increase in non-cardiovascular deaths after more than five years of follow-up. The Multicenter Antiatheroma Study (MAAS) — referenced at the 1994 meeting of the European Society of Cardiology and in the 1994 report in *Circulation* from the Coronary Arteriosclerosis Intervention Trial and in the Canadian Trial — showed no reduction in cardiovascular events. However, none of these studies had the statistical power to do so.

While taking a resounding position in support of secondary prevention, the *BMJ* editorial does point out that the new studies on cholesterol lowering in patients without coronary disease or with already low cholesterol levels do not resolve the issue of possible increase in noncardiac mortality. The editorial also cites the Harvard Atherosclerosis Reversibility Project, reported in 1994 in the *Lancet,* which found that patients who had cholesterol concentrations ranging from approximately 180 to 240 milligrams percent, and who had evidence of mild obstructive coronary disease, did not benefit from three years of statin treatment.

The *BMJ* editorial takes the position that the jury is still out on the benefits of primary prevention, and that conservatism in this area is still justified. But the message is clear and unequivocal that conservatism is no longer acceptable in the treatment of elevated cholesterol concentrations in most patients with coronary disease — that is, after myocardial infarction, after bypass surgery and PTCA — and in those with established coronary artery involvement. The editorial also states that for elderly patients with comorbid conditions that threaten life expectancy, the judgment of the individual physician is still required. In the *European Heart Journal* in 1994, the European Atherosclerosis Society, the European Society of Cardiology and the European Society of Hypertension recommend the use of cholesterol-lowering drugs in patients with cholesterol concentrations over 240 milligrams percent, but only after three to six months of careful dietary counseling has failed. It is axiomatic that in the vast majority of patients, particularly those who are not obese, dietary impact will not be strong. It is also quite evident that the statin drugs reduce cholesterol levels by 25 to 35 percent.

It is significant and interesting that the lead author of the *BMJ* editorial is Michael Oliver. As most of you probably know, Dr. Oliver has been something less than an enthusiast of cholesterol reduction, particularly as primary prevention. It is to his credit that he is now leading the effort to emphasize the risks of high cholesterol in patients with myocardial infarction and in those with established coronary disease. The editorial notes that these admonitions are still ignored to some extent in several European countries, including Britain. The editorial ends with a clear statement that in patients with coronary disease, there is now no justification for inertia in the use of statins.

In the *Lancet* of May 20, 1995, there is a short report titled, "Baseline Serum Cholesterol and Treatment Effect in the 4S Study," written by the authors of that study. They remind us that reduction in the relative risk produced by simvastatin has been shown to be independent of baseline cholesterol levels only for coronary heart disease patients with serum cholesterols in the range of 220 to 320 milligrams percent (or 5.5 to 8 millimols) and with other characteristics similar to the patients studied in the 4S study. The authors suggest further that the extent to which other patients will benefit from cholesterol lowering with statin medications remains to be demonstrated. They refer to the 10-year mortality from cardiovascular disease among patients with lower cholesterol levels, with and without preexisting disease, as reported in the *New England Journal of Medicine* in 1990. They point out that the coronary disease patients with lower cholesterols than those studied in the 4S trial have a better prognosis and may not experience the same absolute reductions in major coronary events as did the 4S patients. The authors of the 4S study add that attempts to explain their results by relating the risk of major coronary events to lipid changes during the trial will require more sophisticated analysis, which they will present in a future report.

While many issues remain in the mystery of atherosclerosis and its prevention and treatment, at this moment, lipid lowering in patients with established coronary disease seems not to be controversial. We have the tools to do the job. It is incumbent on us as cardiologists to lead the way in secondary prevention — or perhaps I should say in secondary treatment — as we have led the way in revascularization. It is also important to remember that any form of revascularization, dramatic and lifesaving as it may be, is really a form of palliation. It is part of the treatment of coronary disease and not an end in itself. This point is brought out very well in an article by James Shepard, one of the authors of the above-discussed *BMJ* editorial. Writing in the *European Heart Journal* in 1995, he says that "coronary heart disease, the single most common cause of debility and death in industrialized countries, is so prevalent that interventional cardiology as currently practiced cannot be expected to have a significant impact on the toll which it exacts from society." Shepard states that "hyperlipidemia warrants such an intervention primarily to cut the risk of cardiovascular disease and minimize coronary morbidity and mortality" — and I'd like to add, especially in those who have had revascularization.

26

The Cholesterol Wars Resume:
Whither Guidelines?

April 1996

Just as it seemed that the cholesterol wars had come to an end, controversy has again erupted, this time from an unlikely source — the American College of Physicians (ACP), in the pages of its journal, the *Annals of Internal Medicine.* A truce, if not peace, in the cholesterol wars was brought about principally by two recent studies. The first of these, the 4S trial, seemed to end all challenge to the use of statins to lower cholesterol for secondary prevention, or perhaps I should say for secondary treatment for patients with known coronary disease. The second report, the West of Scotland Coronary Prevention Study (WO-SCOPS) that used pravastatin, did for primary prevention what the 4S study did for secondary prevention. In an editorial that accompanied the West of Scotland paper, Pederson said, "The benefits of reducing cholesterol were now established beyond any reasonable doubt." The 4S study triggered a marked increase in the use of statins for patients with established coronary disease. In similar manner, the West of Scotland Study produced a sharp rise in the prescription of statins for primary prevention.

It was over this bright and sunny clime that the new ACP guidelines appeared as a dark cloud of controversy. "Guidelines for Using Serum Cholesterol, High-Density Lipoprotein Cholesterol and Triglyceride Levels as Screening Tests for Preventing Coronary Heart Disease in Adults — Part I," an official position paper of the American College of Physicians, was published in the March 1996 issue of the *Annals of Internal Medicine.*

Let's look at these new ACP guidelines. The first of these is that a total cholesterol level is adequate for screening purposes. While a high-density lipoprotein (HDL) level under 35 may be important for risk stratification, its impact on treatment is uncertain and therefore it need not be screened. Triglyceride screening is also omitted because of insufficient evidence that it is a risk factor independent of total and HDL cholesterol. The second is that cholesterol screening be done one time and repeated periodically only if the value is near a treatment threshold. There is little information to help determine precisely how often to screen, but every five years seemed reasonable. The third is that cholesterol screening is not recommended for men under 35 and women under 45 unless there is a familial lipoprotein disorder or at least two other risk factors. The fourth is that cholesterol screening for primary prevention is appropriate but not mandatory for men aged 35 to 65 and women aged 45 to 65. A further caveat from the ACP is that with the "possible exception" (their words) of the recent West of Scotland Study, primary prevention trials have not shown cholesterol reduction to prolong life in middle-aged men with no history of coronary disease. The fifth guideline is that evidence is insufficient to recommend or discourage primary screening in men and women aged 65 to 75. The sixth is that screening is not recommended for men and women aged 75 and older because no clinical trial data are available for this group. And finally, the seventh guideline is that all patients with known coronary disease or a history of other vascular disease should have lipid analyses including, but not necessarily limited to, total cholesterol levels.

Part II of the ACP clinical guidelines, titled, "Cholesterol Screening in Asymptomatic Adults, Revisited," reviews in some detail the documentation, logic and literature to support these new guidelines and is based on pooled analyses of clinical trial data and data from the Framingham Heart Study. The stated conclusion is that cholesterol screening is most likely to be useful when it is done in populations at high, short-term risk of dying from coronary disease, such as survivors of myocardial infarction and middle-aged men with multiple cardiac risk factors. In these populations, cholesterol reduction appears to be both medically useful and cost-effective. In other populations, the benefits are smaller and uncertain.

At what level of risk of death from coronary heart disease do the benefits of therapy outweigh the risks? The ACP authors point out that a therapy that reduces the risk of coronary heart disease by half would reduce the annual mortality from 40 to 20 deaths per 1000 in secondary prevention, but only from four to two deaths per 1000 in primary prevention. Thus a therapy with noncardiac side effects causing two deaths per thousand would still greatly reduce the mortality in secondary prevention but not in primary prevention. The ACP guidelines question the value of screening in the younger age groups and in the elderly. The association between cholesterol level and the risk of coronary artery disease disappears by the late 70s. The guidelines contend that uncertainty of benefit and potential harm from cholesterol lowering is greatest for men and women aged 65 to 75.

In the same issue of the *Annals* there is a perspective by John LaRosa titled, "Cholesterol Agonistes." He disagrees categorically with much that is in the new ACP guidelines, charging that they minimize large elements of data linking cholesterol to atherogenesis and that they make unwarranted and unproved assumptions about physician behavior, in particular, that screening will lead to unnecessary use of lipid-lowering drugs. LaRosa notes that the guidelines purport to promote evidence-based clinical decisions and while that may be a laudable goal, he believes that the ACP over-emphasizes selected epidemiological and clinical trial data and ignores whole categories of important evidence, such as the effect of lipoproteins on vascular wall biology. He also believes that triglyceride screening in selected cases can lead to important interventions. Summing up, LaRosa states that the ACP guidelines are "wrong and misguided."

In a brief editorial entitled, "Evangelists and Snails Redux: The Case of Cholesterol Screening," *Annals* editor, Dr. Frank Davidoff, sees the cholesterol controversy as one that stems from ideological differences between advocates and methodologists (later called evangelists and snails) — terms used in a paper by Sackett and Holland, published in the *Lancet* in 1975. Davidoff believes that primary prevention, unlike secondary screening, is still in the domain of controversy — a shadowy territory where the hard data trail off into uncertainty. He sees the controversy flowing from opposite ends of a single moral question. The evangelists ask, "Isn't it wrong to withhold from patients an intervention with potential benefits and undemonstrated harms?" Whereas the snails ask, "Isn't it wrong to impose on patients an intervention with undemonstrated benefits and potential harms?" While more and better data might sharpen the focus of the cholesterol controversy, even that might be of little help considering that the benefits are relatively infrequent compared to the number of patients treated, the costs of treatment and the possible risks.

Davidoff sees no right or wrong answers in the present cholesterol guidelines controversy. Ultimately, rapprochement must take place on what he calls newly defined common ground, but I'm not certain what he means by "common ground." Perhaps one way to find this common ground is to agree that there are rarely absolutes in medicine and that it is probably not possible for any organization to lay down rigid guidelines for situations that depend on interpretation, judgment and philosophy. In the March 15, 1996 issue of *Circulation*, there is an editorial by the Risk Reduction Task Force of the American Heart Association entitled, "Cholesterol Screening in Asymptomatic Adults: No Cause to Change." While new and convincing evidence such as this would be an impetus to revise the National Cholesterol Education Program/American Heart Association (NCEP/AHA) guidelines, none has been presented by the ACP. Evidence-based guidelines imply a balanced and impartial view of available data, neither of which is represented by the ACP guidelines, according to this editorial.

As I see it, this editorial may be addressing something more important than the issue of cholesterol screening. Perhaps the controversy is really about guidelines. Nothing could bring the fallibility and vulnerability of guidelines more sharply into focus than a careful study of the conflicting ACP and NCEP/AHA positions. The insurance companies, HMOs and even our hospitals, who want blueprints and guidelines for everything a doctor does, must be taken aback a bit by this disagreement and controversy among the experts. After all, what they abhor most is uncertainty and variability in the practice of medicine. Unfortunately, uncertainty and variability are inherent in the practice of medicine.

The American Heart Association and the editorial in *Circulation* express fear that the ACP guidelines are putting practicing physicians in an untenable position because it gives conflicting messages that could cause "professional, legal and financial implications." But conflicting messages may be just what doctors need most because it might force them to study the conflicting data and do some thinking for themselves. Then, based on their own experience and interpretation of data in the literature, they could exercise their clinical judgment — that's what patients go to doctors for in the first place.

27

Aggressive Lipid Lowering — Still Not Aggressively Prescribed

February 1997

The lead article in the January 16, 1997 issue of the *New England Journal of Medicine* continues a veritable flood of recent studies defining and validating the apparent value of lipid lowering for both primary prevention and so-called secondary prevention for patients who have already manifested coronary disease. The article is entitled, "The Effect of Aggressive Lowering of Low-Density Lipoprotein Cholesterol Levels and Low-Dose Anticoagulation on Obstructive Changes in Saphenous-Vein Coronary Artery Bypass Grafts," and it is written by the Post-Coronary Artery Bypass Graft Trial investigators.

In six medical centers in the United States and one in Canada, 1351 patients (of the 2300 screened) enrolled in the study between March 1989 and August 1991. The patients were 92 percent male and 94 percent Caucasian, and their mean age was 61-1/2 years. All of the patients had bypass surgery one to 11 years previously, their LDL cholesterol levels were between 130 and 175 milligrams percent and they had at least one patent graft defined at coronary angiography. The study used a 2 x 2 factorial design with patients assigned to aggressive or moderate LDL lowering, using lovastatin and if necessary, cholestyramine. In addition, some patients received low-dose warfarin or placebo. Angiography was repeated an average of 4.3 years after baseline.

Among the patients whose LDL levels were lowered aggressively (that is, to the 90 milligrams percent range) there was progression of atherosclerosis in 27 percent, versus 39 percent in the group with moderate LDL levels in the 130 milligrams percent range. Revascularization over the 4.3-year period was 6.5 percent in the aggressively treated group and 9.2 percent in the more modestly lowered LDL patients — a difference of 2.7 percent. The low-dose warfarin group attained a mean international normalized ratio of 1.4 and the placebo group had an INR of 1.1. Low-dose warfarin did not influence the progression of atherosclerosis.

In the same issue of the *New England Journal,* an editorial by Valentin Fuster and David Vorchheimer of Mt. Sinai Hospital in New York entitled, "Prevention of Atherosclerosis in Coronary Artery Bypass Grafts," discusses the study just described. The authors remind us that serial angiographic studies show that 15 to 30 percent of vein grafts are stenosed within a year after surgery, nearly 50 percent are closed in 10 years, and some 10 to 20 percent of bypass operations performed in the United States are repeat procedures. Thus, they emphasize the critical importance of long-term approaches to the prevention of graft stenosis after bypass surgery. The results of the study in question — that intensive lipid lowering is of benefit in slowing the progression of obstructive disease in vein grafts after surgery and that low-dose anticoagulation is not of benefit — were of interest to Fuster and Vorchheimer because both lipid deposition and thrombosis appear to be important factors in progression. They note that while rates of progression of atherosclerotic disease and coronary occlusion are reduced by aggressive lipid lowering, no substantial regression in atherosclerotic plaques has been found. They cite their own 1995 *European Heart Journal* paper, which suggests that lipid lowering may tend to stabilize plaques, prevent plaque disruption and slow atherosclerotic progression and occlusion without necessarily reducing plaque size.

The authors postulate that progression of stenosis in native coronary arteries and in bypass grafts is in part related to active mural thrombi at the site of plaque disruption and to myofibrotic nonthrombotic growth that has not yielded to conventional antithrombotic therapy. Secondly, occlusion of native or grafted coronary arteries may be related to the degree of coronary stenosis, to small size, or to low flow in the recipient vessels, causing stasis and fibrin-dependent thrombi that are resistant to both antiplatelet agents and low-dose anticoagulants as used in the current trial. Finally, Fuster and Vorchheimer believe that new antithrombotic strategies deserve to be tested in all phases of coronary disease, including the combination of a platelet inhibitor, such as aspirin or ticlopidine, with moderate-dose anticoagulation, such as oral warfarin with the target INR of 2 to 3, or oral therapy with specific antithrombins and inhibitors of platelet glycoprotein IIb/IIIa receptors.

It should be apparent to anyone observing the clinical scene that while aspirin and other antithrombotic regimens are widely used in patients with coronary disease — and there is some movement toward the use of other antiplatelet agents in combination — the aggressive use of lipid lowering in patients with established coronary disease still lags. This under-utilization of lipid lowering in the United States is documented in a January 1997 paper in the *Journal of the American College of Cardiology* by Stafford, Blumenthal and Pasternak from Massachusetts General Hospital, titled, "Variations in the Cholesterol Management Practices of U.S. Physicians." Stated briefly, the authors found that in some 85 million visits by patients with hyperlipidemia, cholesterol testing was conducted in 23 percent, counseling in 34 percent, and lipid lowering in only 23 percent. The essence of this paper is that American physicians have not yet fully adopted available evidence-based recommendations regarding cholesterol management in patients with hyperlipidemia.

Lipid Modification for Control
of Atherothrombosis

July 1999

The term atherothrombosis has become popular in the literature of cardiology because this single word encompasses the development of the atherosclerotic plaque, its rupture and consequent clot formation, all of which may lead to an unstable coronary syndrome. Atherothrombosis may be asymptomatic or it may cause catastrophic events. The term also epitomizes the major pathological processes involved in ischemic stroke, peripheral vascular disease and coronary syndromes. In the prevention and management of acute coronary syndromes, much attention properly has been paid to antithrombotic and thrombolytic interventions. However, an earlier and very important step in avoiding the sequellae of atherothrombosis may well be aggressive lipid lowering so as to limit the development of the lipid-laden plaque or to cause it to shrink in size by decreasing its highly thrombogenic lipid core.

Pertinent to these discussions there are several papers in the recent medical literature that I believe may be of some interest, depending on the reader's ideas, convictions and prejudices. Perhaps they will also stimulate some thought and even some controversy. The first of these is a paper in the *British Medical Journal* of May 29, 1999 titled, "Why Heart Disease Mortality is Low in France: The Time-Lag Explanation," by Malcolm Law and Nicholas Wald of London. At the outset, the authors quote data on mortality from ischemic heart disease in France, showing that it is about one-fourth of that in Britain. Because major risk factors in France are no more favorable than in Britain and in many other countries, this has been called the "French Paradox." This paradox is often attributed to the higher consumption of alcohol in France — namely of wine and more specifically, red wine. But the authors reject the concept that wine or any kind of alcohol explains the French Paradox because they believe that all alcoholic drinks produce similar changes in HDL cholesterol and hemostatic factors. They cite five large-cohort studies comparing people who drank red wine with those who drank white wine that showed no difference in the incidence of heart disease.

Law and Wald believe that there is a highly significant difference between past and recent fat consumption in France. They contend that in countries with high wine consumption, such as France, Italy, Spain and Switzerland, saturated fat consumption used to be low, but now has increased. They believe that the continued relatively low incidence of coronary disease in France is the result of a time lag — that there may be 25 years or more between an increase in animal fat consumption and changes in cholesterol concentration that would cause coronary atheroma and an increased risk of death from ischemic heart disease. Thus, they suggest that the reduction of heart disease mortality is the result of a time-lag factor rather than the French Paradox based on wine consumption. Incidentally, they also note that the total mortality among British and French men is the same despite a lower mortality from ischemic heart disease in France. In France, the excessive mortality from alcohol-related diseases, such as liver disease, cancels out the relatively low mortality from heart disease. This trend, however, is not found in women whose all-cause mortality in France is one-third less than in Britain. This may be due to moderation of alcohol intake, dietary changes and reduced smoking among French women.

Commenting on this paper, Stanford and Rem from the Brigham and Women's Hospital in Boston say that coronary disease is complex and multifactorial and that this is a good thing because it offers many avenues of intervention. They concede that Law and Wald may well be correct that, in time, the French Paradox will disappear as fat consumption increases in the population. They think that dietary controls have not received adequate attention. Stanford and Rem may be correct in this belief, but while it may be true that dietary fat contributes to the incidence of coronary disease, the success achieved through dietary control alone has not been spectacular. In the July 14, 1999 issue of *European Heart Journal*, there is an article by R. Aquilani from Pavia, Italy and his associates. Its title epitomizes their results: "Despite Good Compliance, Very Little Fat Diet Alone Does Not Achieve Recommended Cholesterol Goals in Out-Patients with Coronary Heart Disease."

Because the relatively recent statin studies have demonstrated that statins are able to reduce LDL cholesterol by some 30 percent or more, it has been widely recognized that statins have a major impact on coronary disease mortality. On the other hand, the effectiveness of interventions to increase HDL and reduce triglycerides has not achieved this degree of acceptance nor perhaps has the effectiveness of the fibrates in this instance been fully validated. In this regard, the VA-HIT trial (Veterans Affairs High-Density Lipoprotein Cholesterol Intervention Trial) may be of some interest and importance. Beginning in 1991, this study took place at 20 VA sites where some 2500 patients were randomized to Gemfibrozil or a placebo. The results of this secondary prevention trial were presented at the 1998 meeting of the American Heart Association. There was a significant reduction in primary coronary heart disease (CHD) endpoints in conjunction with increased high-density lipoprotein (HDL), decreased triglycerides with no change in low-density lipoprotein (LDL) cholesterol.

In the June 1999 issue of *Annales*, a publication of the Royal College of Physicians and Surgeons of Canada, there is a paper entitled, "Cholesterol Revisited: Prime Mover or a Factor in the Progression of Atherosclerosis?" by Sean Moore from McGill University. An accompanying editorial by *Annales* editor, William Feldman, "Cholesterol: Main Culprit or Mere Accomplice?" epitomizes Dr. Moore's thesis that damage to the endothelial lining is the primary event in atherosclerosis and that the deposition of lipid is secondary. Moore contests the idea that hyperlipidemia is the prime mover in atherogenesis, a concept that he claims is based on animal experiments in which high levels of blood lipids were associated with fatty streaks in the arterial intima. He believes that in humans, these fatty streaks are different from the lesions produced in animal experimentation. He also considers that the concept of lipid accumulation in the vessel wall occurring as a result of the trapping of lipoprotein differs fundamentally from the idea that lipoprotein enters the vessel wall in excess amounts because of elevated blood lipoproteins taken up by monocytes to form macrophage foam cells.

Moore notes that in the West of Scotland Study, the absolute reduction of nonfatal and fatal MI was 2.4 percent, meaning that over 200 patients had to be treated for one year to prevent an event. The absolute reduction in mortality was 0.9 percent, requiring 555 men to be treated for one year to prevent one man's death. His conclusion is that these results are not what might be expected if hypercholesterolemia really played the key role in CHD causation and progression. Moore's article is interesting, even if not convincing, and I present excerpts from it here to whet the interest of those who might like to hear what today can only be regarded as an iconoclastic view. It's really not a bad thing to contemplate a contrarian view, even if only to formulate a response or perhaps a refutation. Moore concedes that while lesions do occur in animals subjected to endothelial injury in the absence of hyperlipidemia, high lipids do enhance the process. I think that Moore sets up somewhat of a straw man when he says that preoccupation with elevated cholesterol and hyperlipidemia tends to decrease enthusiasm and interest in researching the cause of atherosclerosis in other areas such as bacteria, viruses and hyperhomocystemia. Perhaps most will agree that there is a tremendous amount of interest in all the factors he mentions and many others, but as yet, none of these avenues of research has negated the primacy of elevated lipids in the genesis of atherosclerosis, at least as we understand it at this time.

A paper to be published in the August 1999 *British Journal of Clinical Practice* by Peter Libby of Boston is titled, "New Insights in Plaque Stabilization by Lipid Lowering." Libby reminds us that the new target is the unstable coronary atheromatous plaque and not the tight stenosis, which up to now has been the traditional focus of interventional cardiology. He refers to the remarkable benefits of lipid-lowering therapy in the reduction of myocardial infarction, sudden death and the reduced need for revascularization. Libby suggests that the benefits of lipid lowering may be partially due to the effect on improved endothelial dilatory function and, on a more chronic time scale, to the reduction of the activation of inflammatory cells. He points to the new therapeutic target — that is, stabilization of the atherosclerotic plaque — that he believes may be more effective in the long run than "bypassing them, squashing them or stenting them." Lipid lowering may yet prove to be more effective in preventing myocardial infarction and in prolonging life than the more dramatic interventional therapies now in vogue.

Cardiovascular Therapeutic Thresholds and Absolute Risk Projection

April 2000

D uring the 1990s, paralleling progress in surgical and catheter-based revascularization, there have been significant advances in understanding the vascular biology and pathology of coronary and systemic cardiovascular syndromes. Medical therapy has become so effective and accepted that comparative revascularization studies are no longer limited to testing only catheter-based versus surgical-based techniques. Today, a growing number of trials compare medical therapy with mechanical forms of revascularization. Beta blockers, angiotensin-converting enzyme inhibitors (ACEIs) and increased understanding of the uses of statins, fibrates and antithrombotic regimens have improved outcomes and contributed to the sophistication of medical approaches.

Prevention and risk factors, much talked about for 50 years, now rightfully command more attention than ever before. This is epito-mized in the *British Medical Journal* of March 11, 2000, a theme issue on risks in cardiovascular disease. The lead editorial in this issue, "Guidelines on Preventing Cardiovascular Disease in Clinical Practice: Absolute Risk Rules Raise Question of Population Screening," is writ-ten by Rodney Jackson, a professor of epidemiology from Auckland, New Zealand. Dr. Jackson's thesis is that 10 years ago, clinical recom-mendations for preventing cardiovascular disease emphasized individ-ual risk factors such as blood pressure and lipids. Separate guidelines based on cohort studies and randomized trials defined methods of management for each of these risk factors and others. Jackson's posi-tion, however, is that over the past decade, there has been a remarkable change from recommendations based on the relative risk imposed by a single risk factor, to recommendations based on absolute risk — in other words, the incidence of cardiovascular events occurring over a specific period of time and based on actual experience. This change in recommendations is based on a synthesis of multiple risk factors. Jeffrey

Rose, arguably the single most influential cardiovascular disease epidemiologist, said in 1991, "All policy decisions should be based on absolute measure of risk; relative risk is strictly for research only." The *BMJ* theme issue brings together several papers that concern what Rodney Jackson calls a paradigm shift in cardiovascular risk management. He cites guidelines that are based on absolute risk that were reported in the *BMJ* by the British Cardiac and Hypertension Societies and the Hyperlipidemia and Diabetic Associations. He also cites similar recommendations that were previously made by the European counterparts of these societies.

Both the British and European societies determine priority for treatment on the absolute risk of events over a defined period of time rather than on what they call the unduly overemphasized relative risk imposed by individual risk factors. In their priorities, the British societies project that the absolute risk of coronary disease over the next 10 years will be in the range of 11 to 30 percent. A 15 percent absolute risk over a decade is considered to be a high risk. Tables show the absolute risk for male and female nonsmokers and smokers aged 34 to 74, with and without diabetes, integrated with systolic blood pressure and with the ratio of serum total cholesterol to HDL cholesterol. The imperative for intervention therefore rests on a single guideline synthesized from several risk factors, rather than on multiple sets of guidelines dealing with each factor individually.

Jackson explains how absolute risk projections would work using data and tables described in another paper in the *BMJ* theme issue entitled, "Updated New Zealand Cardiovascular Risk/Benefit Prediction Guide," which makes a five-year projection. For example, a 50-year-old nonsmoking female with a blood pressure of 170/100, a cholesterol in the range of 240 and an HDL of 48 would have a 6 percent chance of suffering a major cardiovascular event over the next five years; whereas a 60-year-old male smoker with the same blood pressure and the same total cholesterol and an HDL of 40 would have about a 30 percent risk. Appropriate therapy for each of these patients would reduce the projected absolute event rate for the female from 6 to 4 percent — a 2 percent absolute reduction, and for the 60-year-old man, there would be a drop in the projected event rate from 30 to 20 percent — a 10 percent absolute reduction over five years. Another way of putting this is that 50 such women and 10 such men would require five years of treatment to prevent one cardiovascular event.

The concept of absolute risk projection over a period of time is expressed in another paper in the *BMJ* theme issue entitled, "Coronary and Cardiovascular Risk Estimation of Primary Prevention: Validation of a New Sheffield Table in the 1995 Scottish Health Survey," the senior author of which is Erica Wallis. The Sheffield Table reported a 97 percent sensitivity and a 95 percent specificity for coronary risk at 15 percent over 10 years. The predictive value of a negative test was 99.5 percent and for a positive test, it was 73 percent. For a risk of 30 percent over 10 years, the sensitivity was 82 percent and the specificity was 99 percent. The authors conclude that the table identified all patients at high risk for lipid screening, and reduced screening for those at low risk by more than half. This ensures treatment for people at high risk and avoids inappropriate treatment for those at low risk.

Yet another paper in the same *BMJ* issue is "Estimating Cardiovascular Risks for Primary Prevention: Outstanding Questions for Primary Care," written by John Robson from St. Bartholomew's and the Royal London School of Medicine. Like the authors of the other papers to which I have referred, Robson credits the Framingham Heart Study for using combined risk factors to predict the probability of coronary disease. He also describes specific thresholds for treatment. For example, a 30 percent risk of coronary disease over 10 years would identify 3.4 percent of the British population aged 35 to 69 and a further 4.8 percent of this population would be added to the treatment group because of preexisting coronary disease. The annual costs of such treatments are estimated to be £900 million, or nearly $1.5 billion. This threshold has been endorsed by Britain's Department of Health as a reasonable objective. If the threshold for treatment were reduced to 15 percent, it would involve 25 percent of the population and would increase the cost by a factor of three, quite possibly making it cost-prohibitive. Robson argues that the need for evidence and debate is greater where small benefits occur in so large a proportion of the population. He also believes that a debate on policy must include public and primary care and should only be considered together with options for improving nutrition, physical activity and reduction of smoking. He concedes that the evidence for benefit and the "political arithmetic of implementation" is currently somewhat confused in the new guidelines. Robson suggests that it would be unfortunate if treating 25 percent of the population at a 15 percent threshold would deter the treatment of the 10 percent of the population with a 30 percent risk of a coronary event over 10 years. In his editorial, Rodney Jackson supports the idea that high-risk populations be identified first and treated appropriately prior to massive population screening.

A somewhat contradictory view is expressed in an accompanying paper entitled, "Should Treatment Recommendations for Lipid-

Lowering Drugs be Based on Absolute Coronary Risk or on Risk Reduction?" by Dr. Ramachandran and his associates from North Staffordshire Hospital in Stoke-on-Trent. The authors question whether such use of absolute risk might miss the opportunity for prevention in younger patients whose absolute risk threshold for five years is below 15 percent. They contend that this population might gain more from treatment of their main risk factor (for example, hyperlipidemia) when viewed over the context of their greater life expectancy.

In his editorial, Jackson points out that the new Sheffield Table can target patients in need of blood lipid measurements, but this would include almost everyone over age 45. The cost of measuring total and HDL cholesterol in so large a segment of the population would be prohibitive and for this reason is unlikely to occur. As a result, both Jackson and Robson favor screening for those at higher projected risk — in other words, increasing the threshold for screening to maximize the number of events thus prevented. While there may be pragmatic fiscal reasons for this approach, it is not really in keeping with current concerns that the milieu that leads to atherothrombosis begins many years prior to clinical manifestations.

Notwithstanding all that has been said, there are still unsolved problems. While the so-called lifestyle modifications such as healthful diet, control of weight, more exercise and elimination of smoking might be achieved without major fiscal implications, even widespread screening for diabetes, abnormal lipids and elevated blood pressure still appears to be beyond the reach of many highly developed societies. Implementing and maintaining adequate pharmacological prevention and treatment is even more illusive.

While there may be consensus on pharmacological interventions for certain levels of absolute risk, there are still gray areas among relatively younger age groups. Although many of the drugs we use appear to be safe over a period of a decade or more, we really don't know what could result from their use over a period of four or five decades, a situation that may occur if drug treatment were to begin as early as some pathological studies seem to indicate. There are still many risk factors such as hypercoagulability for which there are as yet no practical and clinically applicable approaches to diagnosis, treatment and prevention. Nevertheless, it now seems possible to have a reasonable probability of success in projecting absolute risk over a finite period of years by integrating various risk factors with age and sex. How society chooses to use this knowledge and what resources it is willing to expend to achieve prevention of cardiovascular disease, now perhaps within our reach, remain open questions.

30

The Prevention Paradox

February 1993

S alt restriction in the general population to prevent hypertension is a metaphor for an important philosophic issue in medicine. How far do we go in our advice to the population at large? How far do we go in advising the many to take medicine or change diet or lifestyle to benefit the few? The cholesterol controversy is an obvious parallel to the salt debate.

During the past few days I have been reading a provocative exposition of this subject by Professor Geoffrey Rose, who retired recently from the Chair of Epidemiology at the London School of Hygiene and Tropical Medicine. His book, *The Strategy of Preventive Medicine*, is only 128 pages — my favorite kind of book, one that can be read thoughtfully without loss of sleep, change of lifestyle, or giving up practice. The essence of Rose's message is that to the epidemiologist, the population is the patient and statistics is the measure of success. This contrasts with the physician who treats a person who is already ill or who tries to modify the prognosis in an individual thought to be at high risk.

The book opens with a quotation from Rudolph Virchow, who said that the history of epidemics is the history of disturbances in human culture and from this flows the idea that ultimately, to control a disease one must control the societal factors that give rise to it. Rose describes the prevention paradox, which he defines as preventive measures that bring great benefits to the community, but may offer little to each participating individual. Thus, a person at low risk may derive little benefit from reduction of salt or fat, or modest alcohol intake, but the population at large might benefit a great deal in terms of epidemiological statistics. Rose clearly favors the population rather than the high-risk approach. He epitomizes this when he says that a large number of people exposed to a small risk may generate many more cases than a small number exposed to a high risk. From the point of view of the epidemiologist, where there is mass exposure to risk, even low-level risk, there is need for mass measures of control. Inevitably, this means reducing slight risk in large numbers of people who will gain little bene-fit. Again, the prevention paradox. This is the dilemma we deal with so often in medicine when we try to decide whether to apply epidemio-logical results and standards to the individual patient.

In discussing the limitations of research studies, Rose suggests that the results are expected to be either statistically significant — positive or negative (indicating that a particular exposure does or does not cause a disease) — or not effective. Rose emphasizes, however, that relative risk is not what decision-making is all about. Doubling a trivial risk is still trivial. He asks the question, How low must risk be before it can be regarded as negligible? The concept of negligible benefit is the coun-terpoint to negligible risk. Even for a statistically significant interven-tion, the benefit may be negligible to the individual. Rose concedes that in this dilemma, "the health prize may be the difference between life and death, but if the statistical chance that it will affect a particular in-dividual is too small or remote, then people may not want to bother." As an epidemiologist, Rose drives home his point by saying, "only if [people] choose to bother can prevention really be effective."

I suppose that in treating our patients, each of us has to decide whether the potential risk or benefit is negligible or important. In the final analysis, it is how each of us answers this question that determines which side we take in many therapeutic and diagnostic controversies.

In reaching finite decisions on issues of public health policy, Rose's conclusions are disheartening because public policy depends on knowing the answer to critical questions that are all too often unanswerable. Rose believes that neither the public nor the media has really grasped the fact that some critically important medical and health questions are unan-swerable. Because of this, all of us — including scientific experts and pol-icymakers — have to live with uncertainty. Rose tells it like it is when he says that unfortunately, humankind does bear uncertainty very well.

Geoffrey Rose concludes his book, *The Strategy of Preventive Medi-cine* — which the December 1993 *British Medical Journal* calls his vale-dictory — by saying: "The primary determinants of disease are mainly economic and social and therefore, its remedies must also be economic and social." According to Rose, medicine and politics cannot and should not be kept apart. Whether one chooses Rose's population strategy for prevention or the high-risk approach, is somewhat like the philosophic divide between the politically liberal and the politically conservative. Perhaps the clinician's greatest potential for disservice is to give patients false expectations based on either the population or the high-risk strat-egy without making them aware of the prevention paradox.

31

Observations on the Enigma of Sudden Cardiac Death

February 2000

Sudden cardiac death remains largely unsolved and enigmatic in spite of the advances that have been made in electrophysiology and therapeutics from amiodarone to implantable defibrillators. In the early 1960s, when the introduction of the coronary care unit began the modern era of the management of acute coronary syndromes, Dr. Bernard Lown said that death may be sudden, but it is not unannounced. He was referring to the concept popular at that time that when ventricular ectopy occurred soon after myocardial infarction, it was a harbinger of sudden death and if recognized and treated, it could often prevent death. To some extent this was true, at least in the context of the coronary care unit (CCU) where the treatment at that time was primarily lidocaine, temporary pacing and external defibrillation.

Since then, it has become quite clear that sudden death is all too often unannounced, or if it is announced, we remain incapable of recognizing the announcement. We can, however, define certain categories of patients who are at high risk for sudden cardiac death. Prominent among these are post-myocardial patients with poor left ventricular function and ventricular arrhythmias, patients with various cardiomyopathies and electrophysiological (EP) disturbances (both acquired and congenital) and patients with advanced congestive heart failure. Unfortunately, it is not possible to pinpoint which specific patients in these various groups will ultimately suffer sudden cardiac death. While our present methods of anticipating, preventing and treating cardiac arrest are far better than they were in the early days of coronary care, sudden death is still a major public health problem. The American Heart Association estimates that some 250,000 sudden cardiac deaths occur each year in the United States, but others believe this number is as high as 400,000. Those of us who are more sanguine regarding the progress of cardiology believe that 20 or 30 years ago, this number was half a million or many more. But even if prevention of sudden cardiac death has improved over the past several decades, the extent of this improvement is difficult to define.

At highest risk for sudden cardiac death are those fortunate enough to have had successful resuscitation following cardiac arrest, whether due to ventricular tachyarrhythmias or bradycardias. In these patients, intensive investigation is required, including cardiac catheterization and often EP testing. Intervention may include revascularization and use of various medications, some of which have been shown to reduce the incidence of sudden death, including first, amiodarone, then beta blockers and various antiarrhythmic agents. A meta-analysis published in March 1999 in the *Journal of the American College of Cardiology* found that ACE inhibitors do reduce the risk of sudden death by some 20 percent (a relative number). This is perhaps not surprising in light of the recent Hope Trial which demonstrated that ramopril reduces mortality in patients with vascular disease, hypertension and especially diabetes. But, by all odds, the most compelling advance in the prevention of sudden cardiac death is the implantable cardiac defibrillator (ICD). At the October 1999 meeting of the Canadian Cardiac Society in Quebec City, a consensus conference chaired by Dr. Stuart Connelly of McMaster University in Hamilton stated that he believes that ICDs are superior to drug therapy in preventing sudden cardiac death in survivors of cardiac arrest and that they should be used as first-line treatment.

Last month on ACCEL, Dr. Hein Wellens presented his 30-year perspective on the spectacular advances that have been made in electrophysiology. He was interviewed by Dr. Eric Michelson who said that some 15 or 20 years ago, he would have predicted that our understanding of the basic mechanisms of sudden cardiac death would have given us a much more effective approach to the problem by now. Dr. Wellens responded that, at that time, we probably underestimated the great complexity of what happens in the heart muscle, in a scar and in surrounding tissue. He also made the cogent observation that in the Dutch city of Maastricht where he works, only 10 percent of the people who experience sudden cardiac death outside the hospital would be categorized as a high risk had there been the opportunity to examine them. Wellens added that many of these patients died from plaque rupture that occurred in only moderately stenotic lesions that had not produced symptoms. This adds to our understanding of why it is so difficult, if not impossible, to anticipate sudden death in large segments of the population.

Against all these odds, efforts continue to close the gap in our ability to anticipate sudden cardiac death. In April 1999, the FDA approved a noninvasive test to improve the ability to predict sudden arrhythmic cardiac death. It was developed by Dr. Richard Cohn of the Harvard-MIT Division of Health Sciences and Technology. The device measures T-wave alternans during exercise stress — changes so small they cannot be detected by the standard electrocardiogram. The ultimate value and applicability of this technology, however, has yet to be proved.

In sudden cardiac death, as in all conditions that elude definitive diagnosis and treatment, it is astounding how many remedies are introduced. For example, the Harvard Physicians Health Study, which followed more than 21,000 men for 12 years, concluded that two to four alcoholic drinks per week reduce the risk of cardiac death by approximately 60 percent and that five or six drinks a week reduce risk by 79 percent (I assume these are relative reductions). Even eating fish has been said to reduce the risk of sudden cardiac death.

Unfortunately, the clearly life-saving ICD is not applicable to the vast majority of patients who ultimately experience sudden cardiac death. While we can define certain groups that are highly susceptible to sudden death, we cannot select the specific patients within these groups in whom sudden death will occur. Thus far, our efforts at prevention have failed to protect most of these people. Even more frightening is the fact that thousands experience sudden death without exhibiting any prior symptoms and without our knowledge that disease even existed. For all too many, death is indeed not only sudden, but unannounced.

32

New Medicine from Old: Hirudin and the Leech

October 1992

In any discussion of thrombolysis, the mention of heparin as an adjunct is inevitable. There is also a continuing search for an antithrombotic agent that is superior to heparin. This prompted me to look at the origins of one of these possibilities — hirudin. It is strange indeed that hirudin — now made available by recombinant DNA technology, that most modern of methodologies — derives from one of medicine's most ancient therapeutic agents, the leech.

In an article in the *Annals of Internal Medicine* of September 1, 1988, Steven Adams, from my own alma mater, Northwestern, writes on the medicinal leech. He describes the ancient uses of and legends surrounding leeches and how their history has been inexorably associated with that of the physician. Even the word "leech" may very well have come from the old English "laece," meaning physician. Adams adds a bit of trivia that might be welcome to many present-day critics of doctors. Long ago, Anglo-Saxon practitioners of medicine and magic were often referred to as leeches.

In the long history of blood-letting in medicine, leeches were used when local rather than systemic bleeding was needed. There were many uses of leeches, including for hemorrhoidal tumors, for epididymitis in which the leeches were applied over the spermatic cord, and for ocular inflammation in which the leeches were placed over the temporal areas. In the first third of the 19th century, five to six million leeches were used annually in Parisian hospitals and as many as 30 million leeches a year were imported to the United States from Germany. At one point, the leech even became considered an endangered species. The leech most commonly used for medicinal purposes is *Hirudo medicinalis*, a freshwater creature about 10 centimeters long that sucks blood through contractions of its muscular pharynx. It has the ability to ingest 10 times its own weight in blood.

Hirudin was first described in 1884 as an anticoagulant secreted by the medicinal leech. It is a polypeptide with an affinity for thrombin. Hirudin inhibits the thrombin-catalyzed conversion of fibrinogen to fibrin. The leech also secretes hyaluronidase and a vasodilator in the form of an antihistamine. Leeches are still used today for repairing grafted skin flaps, for digital reimplantations and breast reconstruction and occasionally, for evacuating periorbital hematomas. There is an article titled, "Hirudin and Derivatives as Anticoagulant Agents," by F. Markwardt in a 1991 issue of the journal, *Thrombosis and Haemostasis*, that elucidates the action of hirudin and tells how through recombinant DNA technology, a number of hirudins similar to the natural substance have been produced on so large a scale that widespread clinical trials are now possible.

Hirudin is also an effective antithrombotic agent in antithrombin III-depleted individuals and because it exerts no influence on platelet formation, it can be used in conditions where quantitative defects of heparin-induced thrombocytopenia may present a risk. Anyone who has ever dealt with the complications of heparin-induced thrombocytopenia will especially appreciate the prospect of an alternative to heparin. An editorial in the September 5, 1992 issue of the *Lancet* entitled, "Hirudins: Return of the Leech," suggests that hirudins may be a more effective anticoagulant than heparin in arterial thrombosis, including thrombosis after angioplasty or thrombolytic therapy, and in the prevention of thrombosis during hemodialysis or cardiopulmonary bypass.

If you think that the use of hirudin in the treatment of coronary thrombosis or intravascular coagulation is new, you should consult the article in the *Journal of the Mt. Sinai Hospital* entitled, "Coronary Thrombosis: Proposed Treatment by Hirudin," written in 1943 by Dr. Howard Lilienthal. Dr. Lilienthal cites the use of leeches in early thrombophlebitis of the lower extremity with the leech being placed over neighboring tissue and not over the vessel. After the animal relaxes its hold and is removed, recovery is often rapid with loss of pain and swelling and full ambulation in less than a week. Dr. Lilienthal quite astutely attributed this favorable effect to hirudin remaining in the body after the leech was removed.

Lilienthal was actually seeking a treatment for coronary thrombosis, which in 1943, according to data quoted from the Metropolitan Life Insurance Company, ranked third as a cause of death, exceeded only by cancer and other disorders of the heart. Lilienthal cites a symposium on coronary thrombosis published in the *Proceedings of the Staff Meetings of the Mayo Clinic* in 1942, in which a paper on management advised only rest, analgesics and sedation.

But Lilienthal does mention that until "recently" (remember, he was writing in 1943), other treatments for coronary thrombosis had included blood-letting using leeches. As already noted, he knew that the value of the leech was not sucking blood, but the hirudin it left in the patient's body after the leech was removed. While Lilienthal could find nothing in the literature to support the use of hirudin to treat intravascular coagulation, he was aware the hirudin could dissolve unorganized intravascular clots. While Lilienthal found interest but not cooperation from fellow physicians for using anticoagulant treatment, he noted that surgeons were more receptive than internists or general practitioners. He quoted a letter that he had received from Dr. Alton Ochsner of Tulane who said, "I have tried to get my medical friends interested in using leeches in coronary thrombosis and have told them that if I ever develop [the disease], I want them to cover me with leeches because I am thoroughly convinced that hirudin is a potent drug and would be of benefit in some cases."

Lilienthal was prophetic when he said that hirudin can do no harm and may turn out to be an advancement in the care of coronary thrombosis. He felt it would be unfortunate to leave therapeutic experiments with hirudin to future generations. He was correct that anticoagulants would be important in the treatment of coronary thrombosis, just as he was correct that the therapeutic experiments with hirudin would be left to future generations. As it turns out, we are one of those future generations.

As a postscript, two months after this editorial appeared, I received a letter from John Horgan of Dublin, who has been an ACCEL guest on more than one occasion. He wrote, "I enjoyed your discussion on leeches, particularly the relevance of the term 'leech' which is used to describe a doctor in English. You will be interested to know that the Irish name, O'Higgins, with which you're probably familiar, means 'grandson of a leech,' the Irish word 'Uigginn' meaning a leech. The O'Higginses were physicians in the old Gaelic clan system which existed up to about the year 1500." John Horgan closes with the comment, "As you are well aware, there is nothing new under the sun."

33

Anticoagulation Therapy After Myocardial Infarction: The More Things Change . . .

April 1995

"Costs and the Effects of Long-Term Oral Anticoagulant Treatment After Myocardial Infarction" is the title of a March 1995 article in the *Journal of the American Medical Association* by the investigators at the ASPECT Coordinating Center at Erasmus University in the Netherlands. (ASPECT stands for anticoagulants in the secondary prevention of events in coronary thrombosis.) An earlier study from the ASPECT investigators that appeared in the *Lancet* in 1994, provided the data for evaluating the economic impact of anticoagulants on post-myocardial infarction.

ASPECT was a placebo-controlled, double-blind, multicenter study conducted in some 60 hospitals in the Netherlands. Patients were randomized to either anticoagulants or placebo. The mean follow-up was 37 months in an overall range of 6 to 76 months. There were some 1700 patients in each group with 170 deaths in the anticoagulant group and 189 deaths in the placebo group. In the anticoagulant group, there were 114 recurrent myocardial infarctions and 242 in the placebo group. The placebo patients also had more acute angiography and angioplasty. During the mean 37-month follow-up period, the placebo patients had approximately 3700 more hospital days than the anticoagulant patients — 2000 days of which were for acute MI and 1000 of which were for unstable angina. The total cost for the anticoagulant patients was 1.5 million Dutch guilders less than for the placebo group (about $900,000). A more clinically compelling study would have been a comparison between aspirin and anticoagulants for both medical and economic outcomes. The authors concede that their study was flawed because it did not make this comparison.

In the same issue of *JAMA*, there is an editorial on the economics and efficacy of using oral anticoagulants versus aspirin after MI, written by John Cairns and Barbara Markham from McMaster University in Hamilton, Ontario. They remind us that oral anticoagulants for the long-term treatment of post-myocardial infarction are more frequently used in Europe than in North America. In a study on long-term anti-coagulants after MI published in the *American Heart Journal* in 1985, Goldberg, Gore, Dalen and Alpert found that in the 1970s, 60 percent of coronary care unit directors in Europe advocated chronic long-term anticoagulation compared with only 3 percent in the United States and none in Britain. The authors were skeptical that anticoagulation after MI decreased the rate of reinfarction or late mortality. The Cairns and Markham editorial cites 1970 and 1980 reviews in the *Lancet* that favor anticoagulants after myocardial infarction, but again the comparison was with placebo.

A 1980 German-Austrian trial that compared aspirin with antico-agulants in some 900 patients yielded nonsignificant results. The 1982 French EPSIM study, reported in the *New England Journal of Medicine*, found a 10.3 percent long-term mortality for anticoagulation and an 11.1 percent mortality for aspirin, but this study may have been pre-maturely stopped. Two studies now in progress comparing warfarin and aspirin — the Coumadin Aspirin Reinfarction Study (CARS) and the Combination Hemotherapy and Mortality Prevention Study (CHAMPS) — may ultimately solve the dilemma of whether to use anticoagulants or aspirin in long-term post-MI care. An interesting sidebar to the ASPECT studies, and to the other articles mentioned above, is that none of them gives the reader a sense of the history of an-ticoagulant therapy, which dates back to the late 1940s, or a sense of the controversy that exists on the best long-term treatment of patients after myocardial infarction.

In his preliminary report in the *American Heart Journal* in 1946, Irving S. Wright advocated the use of dicumarol in all cases of coro-nary thrombosis and he proposed the need for a more extensive study. Such a study was started that same year under the auspices of the American Heart Association and the U.S. Public Health Service. It was one of the first major multicenter trials in cardiology. There were 16 participating hospitals, some of the more famous of which included Beth Israel in Boston, Cincinnati General, Mount Zion in San Fran-cisco, Peter Bent Brigham in Boston, Jackson Memorial in Miami, Michael Reese in Chicago and of course, New York Hospital, where Irving Wright worked. Some of the more famous investigators in-cluded Johnson McGuire, Herman Blumgart, Louis Katz, Herman Hellerstein, Samuel Levine, Sterling Nichol and John Sampson. Inci-dentally, I was an intern at Michael Reese at the time and observed this study first-hand.

In 1948, Wright reported favorably in *JAMA* on the first 1800 cases from this study. Randomization at the time was very simple: admissions on odd days were treated with anticoagulants and admissions on even days were given conventional therapy. Twenty-four percent of the control patients died during hospitalization compared to a 15 percent mortality in the patients who received oral anticoagulants. Aside from the reduction in mortality of 9 per 100 patients in the treated group, these data are a staggering reminder of the high mortality from acute myocardial infarction at the time when this study was done. Thromboembolic events occurred in 25 percent of the controls and in 11 percent of anticoagulant-treated patients.

In the June 1954 issue of *Circulation*, Tulloch and Wright reported on the favorable results of using anticoagulant therapy for seven years after MI. Four years later, Sterling Nichol, one of the pioneers in long-term post-MI anticoagulation, reported on the results from 10 institutions. In 1000 cases, the two-year mortality was 12 percent for those given anticoagulant therapy and 28 percent for those not given anticoagulants. One of the authors of this study was the late George Griffith of Los Angeles, who many of you know as an important figure in the history of the American College of Cardiology. In 1956, Keyes, Drake and Smith reported in *Circulation* on what they called the "unequivocal proof" of increased MI survival with long-term anticoagulant therapy. But again, this was a study involving anticoagulants versus placebo instead of aspirin, which was not yet being used for post-myocardial infarction patients.

The paper that may best put the history of anticoagulation in myocardial infarction in perspective was written by the late Arthur Selzer of San Francisco, with whom I once had the pleasure of spending a month's sabbatical. In the June 1978 issue of the *American Journal of Cardiology* (which at the time was called the *Journal of the American College of Cardiology*), Selzer said that since 1946, the use of anticoagulant therapy in acute MI has been the subject of one of the liveliest controversies in clinical medicine. In his incisive and perhaps iconoclastic manner, Selzer analyzed these studies on post-MI anticoagulation from the point of view of design, reliability and clinical relevance. He found an overemphasis on design and reliability and a singular lack of concern for clinical relevance. Selzer also commented on the "statistically significant differences" which he believed by then had become a part of the daily vocabulary of physicians. He questioned whether this trend had led to an over-reliance on and a misinterpretation of the concept of statistical significance — a question that is still often raised. Selzer reviewed 32 studies comparing anticoagulants with placebo after acute

MI and found that the results ranged from a 2.5-fold reduction in mortality to no change at all.

Rightly or wrongly, Selzer reasoned that the benefits of anticoagulation after myocardial infarction were related to early ambulation, which eliminates thromboembolic complications, and that attributing the reduction in mortality to anticoagulants was untenable and extravagant. He believed this in spite of the fact that in 1946, when it was shown that thromboembolic events were reduced, the treatment for MI was six weeks of immobilization in bed. Lost in much of Selzer's discussion is the fact that from the 1950s through the 1970s and beyond, long-term anticoagulant therapy after myocardial infarction enjoyed a considerable vogue.

Just this week, I saw a patient from another city who, after having been on continuous warfarin therapy since he suffered an anterior wall myocardial infarction in 1965, finally required bypass surgery for symptomatic triple-vessel disease. There are many such anecdotal experiences that in retrospect might support the use of long-term warfarin therapy after infarction, especially when we recall that at the time, aspirin was not in the equation. Still the controversy goes on — "the more things change...."

I would like to add one final observation on the ASPECT paper and the economic impact of anticoagulants after myocardial infarction. If indeed it turns out that anticoagulants after MI are better than antiplatelet therapy, who is to say that this treatment should not be used even if it is more expensive? And to take the matter a step further, who is to decide at what level of increased cost an effective and perhaps lifesaving therapy should be considered economically contraindicated? In the long run, this question may prove more difficult to answer than whether long-term anticoagulant therapy is superior to antiplatelet therapy — a consideration that may apply to many of the therapeutic interventions that we analyze so assiduously. The definition of cost-effectiveness may be more elusive than many would have us believe.

34

Coronary Angiography:
Controversy Over Indications

January 1993

I can't resist saying a few words about a paper that has recently received a great deal of coverage in the press and which could end up having a considerable impact on the practice of cardiology if the results presented and the conclusions of the authors are taken seriously. I am referring to the paper in the November 11, 1992 issue of the *Journal of the American Medical Association* titled, "Results of a Second Opinion Trial Among Patients Recommended for Coronary Angiography," by Graboys, Biegelson, Lampert, Blatt and Lown.

The study is based on a cohort of 171 patients with coronary artery disease who were referred to the Lown group for a second opinion prior to scheduled or recommended coronary angiography. Of this group, 76 percent were self-referred or were referred by the suggestion of a family member and 24 percent were referred by a physician or by an insurance carrier who wanted a second opinion. Because three patients were lost to follow-up, the study ultimately consisted of 168 patients. Of these, 134 (80 percent) did not meet the Lown group criteria for angiography. A decision was deferred in 28 patients (16 percent) pending further studies and there was confirmation of the previous recommendation for coronary angiography in only six patients (4 percent) of the original cohort. Of the 28 patients who were reevaluated, only three were recommended for angiography and the remaining 25 were placed on a modified medical regimen. Thus, of the 168 patients who had originally been advised to have coronary angiography, only nine were so advised by the Lown group. The follow-up period was a mean of 46.5 months.

The authors make a sweeping statement: "We reasonably conclude that an estimated 50 percent of coronary angiography currently being undertaken in the United States is unnecessary or at least could have been postponed." They do concede that "there may be a limitation in terms of generalizing this experience to all patients with coronary disease." During the 46.5-month follow-up period, there were 11 deaths, 7 of them cardiac, which the authors annualized to a mortality of 1.1 percent; 19 patients had myocardial infarction for an annual rate of 2.7 percent; 127 developed unstable angina, annualized at 4.3 percent; and 26 patients (15.4 percent) ultimately had coronary bypass surgery or angioplasty. The annualized event rate for death, myocardial infarction and new-onset unstable angina may seem insignificant in the way it was presented by the authors, but when totaled, 53 patients, or nearly one-third of the cohort, died or had myocardial infarction or developed new-onset unstable angina. I would hardly consider this to be a favorable result or a reason to make the given claim against coronary angiography.

The disquieting thing about this study is the wide publicity given to the authors' conclusion that 50 percent of coronary angiograms in the United States are unnecessary or should be postponed. Because the paper was published in *JAMA*, it received very wide attention indeed. A headline in the *Wall Street Journal* for November 11, 1992 read: "Heart Study Calls Angiograms Overused by 50 Percent — Other Doctors Dispute Results." The *New York Times* ran the headline: "Study Sees Excess in X-Rays of Heart — 50 Percent of Coronary Angiograms are Called Unnecessary — Conclusions Disputed." *USA Today* declared: "Heart Catheter Test May Be Overused" and the *Washington Post* reported: "Heart Disease X-Rays Seen as Overused — Study Says 500,000 Costly Angiograms a Year May Be Unnecessary."

A headline in the *Medical Tribune* of December 10, 1992 reads: "Top Cardiologists Rap Study on Angiography Overuse." The article quotes Rene Favaloro, formerly of the Cleveland Clinic and now Director of the Institute of Cardiology and Cardiovascular Surgery in Buenos Aires: "I am really mad with some of the big journals in this country," he says. "The editorial board should be more careful about reading and analyzing these papers before they publish them. You cannot make these calculations on such a small number of patients." Favaloro concedes that some people are doing unnecessary cineangiograms for the money, as he puts it, but this cannot be extrapolated to the whole field of cardiology. Eric Topol of the Cleveland Clinic Foundation is also quoted as saying that the answer can come only with a study in which half the patients are catheterized and the other half not catheterized. He notes that the Lown group reported an observational study in a small and skewed sample. Topol calls the authors' broad extrapolations "unreasonable." Dolph Hutter, President of the American College of Cardiology, who also disputes the study, is quoted by the *New York Times* as saying that the findings cannot be extrapolated as the authors did to all the coronary angiograms done in this country.

I do not think any experienced cardiologist would deny that there are some excesses and extravagances in coronary angiography. But to say, on the basis of a small observational study of a highly selected group of patients, that 50 percent of the coronary angiograms in the United States are unnecessary or could be delayed is a highly subjective and questionable conclusion. It might be acceptable to offer such a subjective impression in an editorial, but to publish this conclusion as the valid result of a scientific study in a leading medical journal is unfortunate. Although the paper has already received a great deal more publicity than it deserves, I think it important to speak out against the sweeping conclusions that the authors have made from a seriously flawed study. I would really like to hear what our ACCEL listeners think.

An Update: March 1993

I received quite a bit of feedback from listeners who wrote to me in response to my request for opinions on the Lown group's conclusion about unnecessary angiograms. Clearly, there is widespread interest in this matter.

Dr. Thomas LaMattina, a practicing cardiologist from Tufts Medical School, writes, "I want you to know that I agree wholeheartedly with your remarks. I am quite disturbed that this publication came out and even more upset regarding the amount of attention it received from the lay press." Dr. LaMattina is sharply critical of ABC World News and Channel 5 in Boston for promoting the article as news and in his opinion, misleading the public.

Dr. Daniel C. Brown of Billingham, Washington, criticizes *JAMA* for even publishing the paper. Dr. Edward Williams of Westfield, New Jersey; Michael Rabbino of San Mateo, California; Carl Chelius of Cudahy, Wisconsin and Ronald Rubinstein of Neptune, New Jersey, among others, oppose the Lown group's conclusions. Richard Kirkpatrick of Longview, Washington, writes that he does not disagree with the position taken by these investigators, but he believes that the problem does not relate to the integrity of cardiologists, but to the inaccuracy of noninvasive strategies for defining coronary disease.

A letter from Dr. Graboys, one of the authors, steadfastly defends his position, stating that his paper has prompted both medical and lay communities to ask a number of fundamental questions about the large number of cardiovascular interventions in this country. He reports having received hundreds of letters from physicians who support his views. According to Dr. Graboys, "It is clear that the majority of individuals with coronary disease and intact left ventricular function can be managed medically with an excellent quality of life. This is precisely the group of individuals who are being subjected to coronary angiography. One might ask what are the nonclinical factors responsible for this glut of intervention?" He answers his own question: "Economic incentives, over-training of interventional subspecialists, and the public and press perception that this is a 'fix-it' problem."

In my commentary, I said that there are some cases of excessive use and extravagances in coronary angiography. Graboys quite agrees and he asks why there has not been a study addressing this problem. My answer is that there are accepted standards for identifying indications for coronary angiography, for example, the guidelines promulgated by the American Heart Association and the American College of Cardiology. Thus far, neither guidelines nor clinical trials nor randomized mega-trials have removed controversy from medical decision-making. This is in large measure because of continuing differences in interpretation of both guidelines and clinical trials. This is not necessarily a bad thing; if it were, the practice of medicine would cease to be the changing, dynamic institution that it is. And speaking of controversy, it is interesting that in 1991, Graboys and Lown were part of a televised discussion on "The Benign Nature of Coronary Disease."

In the February 10, 1993 issue of *JAMA*, there is a paper related to the current controversy entitled, "Appropriateness of the Use of Coronary Angiography in New York State." Conducted by the Rand Corporation with the participation of UCLA, Michigan State and Harvard, it is a retrospective review of some 1300 patients who underwent coronary angiography in 1990 in 15 randomly selected hospitals. Using a modified Delphi Technique, a nine-member expert panel rendered a retrospective judgment of appropriateness based on 2100 possible indications in 10 clinical categories. The result was that 75 percent of the angiograms were rated appropriate, 20 percent were rated uncertain and only 4 percent were considered inappropriate. This is in sharp contrast to the 50 percent of unnecessary angiograms claimed by Lown and his co-authors.

The Rand Corporation is not known to be overly generous in its appraisal of the appropriateness of interventions by physicians. In 1988, *JAMA* published a Rand appropriateness study on coronary artery bypass surgery that found 56 percent appropriate, 30 percent equivocal and 14 percent inappropriate. But by 1993, in the same journal, a paper from Rand on bypass surgery presented entirely different results: 91 percent were appropriate, 7 percent uncertain and only 2.4 percent inappropriate. Thus between 1988 and 1993, successive publications from the Rand Corporation show a striking difference in the incidence of inappropriate bypass surgery. Their study on PTCA in New York state reports 58 percent appropriate, 38 percent uncertain and 4 percent inappropriate. These three recent Rand studies contradict the data and views of Lown's group that we are pursuing massively unnecessary interventions in cardiology, including angiography, PTCA and bypass surgery.

35

On the Virtues of a Normal Coronary Angiogram: Clinical and Economic

July 1996

In the June 1996 issue of *Heart*, there is a paper from the Department of Cardiology of Glenfield General Hospital, in Leicester, England, with the intriguing title: "Normal Coronary Angiograms: Financial Victory from the Brink of Clinical Defeat?" At issue are the questions of when to do coronary angiography, what are the most valid indications and what noninvasive strategies may obviate the necessity for angiography in patients with chest pain syndromes. This paper makes the observation that "a normal coronary angiogram is sometimes interpreted as a failure of a pre-procedural evaluation, an unnecessary risk to the patient and a waste of scarce resources. It is possible, however, that the diagnostic precision offered by knowledge of the coronary anatomy has benefits in terms of illness behavior and health care resource consumption that far outweigh the cost of angiography."

The authors' stated objective is to examine the hypothesis that a normal angiogram results in a reduction of subsequent healthcare expenses for patients undergoing angiography for suspected coronary disease. A retrospective cost/benefit analysis comparing the 12-month period before and after angiography was carried out in a tertiary cardiac referral center. The study involved 69 consecutive patients with normal angiograms who were investigated in 1991 and 1992. The medical costs included hospital admissions, drugs prescribed in the 12 months before and after angiography, consultations and visits to general practitioners — in other words, all expenses incurred in the evaluation of chest pain symptoms. The mean cost of care for patients with normal angiograms during the year before the investigation was about £650, or roughly $1000. The decrease in medical expenditures following a normal angiogram was approximately $55 a month. Thus the authors estimate that the cost of performing the angiogram would be recouped in about 18 months.

The 69 patients with normal angiograms represented only 8 percent of diagnostic catheterizations during the time of the Leicester study. The 49 percent of patients with normal angiograms had a positive stress test and 25 percent had a negative one. The other 25 percent had no precatherization stress test. Of the 69 patients, there was no procedure-related morbidity or mortality, but one death did occur suddenly during the following year. There were no necropsy data. In spite of the reduced cost of caring for patients with chest pain syndromes during the year following a normal angiogram, only 53 percent of general practitioners reported that the normal angiogram made the management of their patients any easier. This illustrates the continued morbidity and symptoms experienced by many patients with chest pain syndromes and normal angiograms.

In the presence of a normal angiogram, chest pain simulating cardiac disease may be due to both cardiac and noncardiac causes. The literature states that patients with chest pain and normal angiograms have a 98 percent 7- to 10-year survival rate. Patients with persistent symptoms, thought to be due to cardiac disease, are usually classified as having syndrome X, still a poorly understood entity. However, as is the case with most cardiac units, the Leicester group did not pursue systematic investigation of noncardiac causes of chest pain following normal angiograms. This was left to the primary care or referring physicians who, in 75 percent of cases, did not carry out further studies. The inference is that the exclusion of obstructive coronary disease with its favorable long-term prognosis tends to deter the continued investigation of chest pain.

A potential limitation of the Leicester study, as suggested by the authors themselves, is the extent to which their results can be generalized to patients presenting with unexplained chest pain. The patients in this study were highly selected in that their clinical and noninvasive evaluation had determined at least a moderate prior probability of coronary disease. This is supported by the fact that only 8 percent of the studied patients had normal angiograms, while the data generally quoted in the literature suggest that in many laboratories, the normal angiogram rate is from 5 to 30 percent, although 30 percent would be high.

This study should not be interpreted as a license to use coronary angiography indiscriminately as a substitute for thoughtful, clinical and noninvasive evaluation. It does, however, imply that patients with a reasonable probability of coronary disease, especially those requiring multiple medications and repeated medical encounters, may benefit both symptomatically and economically from definition of the coronary anatomy. If case selection for coronary angiography is indeed scrupulous, a normal study does not mean improper utilization, nor is it necessarily profligate of medical resources. Quite to the contrary, it may be highly cost-effective.

The results of this unique study may give some perspective when considering indications for coronary angiography and the cost-effectiveness of diagnostic strategies emphasizing a noninvasive approach for patients with equivocal chest pain. Perhaps there are some occasions when the angiographic option can be chosen before doctors, patients and pocketbooks are exhausted by the now burgeoning inventory of noninvasive technologies.

36

Toward a Definition of
Myocardial Ischemia

February 1995

In the December 1994 issue of *Cardiovascular Research*, there is an editorial that asks an intriguing question in its title: "Myocardial Ischaemia: Can We Agree on a Definition for the 21st Century?" The editor-in-chief of *Cardiovascular Research*, David Hearse, sought to answer this question by requesting a simple definition of ischemia from 33 eminent cardiologists — individuals "who have earned their living at least in part from ischemia." Hearse reports that the responses he received confirm that there is no clear universal definition of myocardial ischemia but that they reveal a number of interesting concepts and caveats.

There was a 94 percent response to Hearse's question and he left it up to the readers to guess who the two eminent cardiologists were who failed to respond in spite of several reminders. Each participant was asked for one short paragraph. The results ranged from three words from Heinrich Shelbert, who defined ischemia as supply-demand imbalance, to a 404-word answer from Jennings and Reimer. Arnold Katz expressed his definition simply: "blood supply inadequate to meet the energy needs of the heart." Gerd Heusch defined ischemia as reduction of blood flow with functional or metabolic consequences. Eric Feigl described it as a restriction of coronary blood flow with pathological alterations of contractile, electrical or biochemical function. Others, such as Julian Hoffman, went into greater detail, mentioning cytokines and alterations in cardiac genes and gene products. Jennings and Reimer talked about a shift in intracellular energy metabolism from aerobic respiration to anaerobic glycolysis.

Hearse chided some of the respondents such as Shelbert, Katz, Willerson, Hoffman and Ruigrok, for taking anthropomorphic liberties with regard to the myocardium and its intentions. He argued that the heart demands nothing, it simply responds in an appropriate manner to the nutritional and neurohormonal milieu in which it exists.

At best, I can only give you a sense of this unique, provocative and somewhat satirical discussion that is spread over 10 pages. As Hearse suggests, there are some contradictions, such as Robert Kloner's contention that ischemia is a reduction in blood flow to the point where myocardial metabolism shifts from aerobic to anaerobic. By this definition, the hibernating myocardium — which does not produce lactate, metabolize substrates oxidatively and has no significant depletion of adenosine triphosphase or creatine phosphate — is clearly not ischemic. In contrast, according to the definition given by John Ross in which ischemia requires a reduction in myocardial blood flow sufficient to cause a decrease in myocardial contraction, the hibernating myocardium would be clearly ischemic.

Suffice it to say that the results of this exercise show that there is no universally accepted definition of myocardial ischemia. This is probably just the problem Hearse was grappling with when he thought to seek help from experts by asking them for their definitions. When all is said and done, cardiologists seeking to define ischemia may have the same problem that legislators have in defining pornography. It is hard to define, but they know it when they see it. Perhaps we should consider the response of Philip Poole-Wilson who, in his response to Hearse, wrote that cardiovascular scientists and clinicians seeking to define ischemia might well heed the words of philosopher Ludwig Wittgenstein: "When one doesn't know what to say, it's best to remain silent." Poole-Wilson concedes, however, that it is unlikely that those who submitted definitions will accept this view.

37

Inflammation, Infection and Acute Coronary Disease

April 1999

There is an article in the April 1999 *European Heart Journal* entitled, "Inflammatory Status as a Main Determinant of Outcome in Patients with Unstable Angina, Independent of Coagulation Activation and Endothelial Cell Function," by M.F. Verheggen and six associates from Leiden University in the Netherlands. Although inflammation, endothelial cell function and the coagulation system are involved in the onset and course of unstable angina, the authors point out that whether a proinflammatory state independently determines outcome is unknown. They present data from a prospective study of markers of inflammation, coagulation activity and endothelial cell function in consecutive patients with unstable angina. Inclusion criteria were typical angina at rest lasting less than 30 minutes within the 24-hour period following admission, in combination with electrocardiographic evidence of myocardial ischemia, prior Q-wave myocardial infarction or coronary angiography that showed at least a 50 percent lumenal narrowing in one large epicardial artery. All patients, unless contraindicated, received aspirin, nitroglycerine and a heparin infusion. Beta and calcium blockers were used at the discretion of attending physicians. The endpoint of the study was refractory unstable angina, which was defined by the need for urgent angiography in spite of optimal medical treatment. This was a decision made by the attending cardiologist without knowledge of the markers of inflammation, which included C-reactive protein (CRP), fibrinogen levels and sedimentation rate.

The 294 patients with unstable angina were admitted to the hospital over an 18-month period. Exclusions because of intercurrent inflammatory or neoplastic disease or absence of ST-T segment criteria or informed consent reduced the study to 211 patients, 150 of whom were men aged 33 to 85 years, with a mean age of 63. The hospital stay

lasted up to 26 days with a mean stay of 4.7 days. The endpoint of refractory unstable angina requiring coronary angiography occurred in 76
patients of whom 6 died of cardiac causes, 10 had an acute inhospital
myocardial infarction and 63 had emergency PTCA or bypass surgery.
The remaining 135 patients (64 percent of the study) remained free of
symptoms with only medical therapy. No inhospital myocardial infarction, cardiac death or urgent revascularization occurred in this group.
CRP, fibrinogen and sedimentation rate were significantly higher in
patients in whom refractory unstable angina occurred than in patients
who could be stabilized by medical means. The relationship of inflammatory markers to poor outcome was not affected by the presence or
absence of myocardial necrosis as indicated by troponin-T levels. There
was no association of markers of coagulation activation or of endothelial dysfunction with inhospital outcome.

These results suggest that an increase in inflammatory activity re-
flects the severity of the underlying process and determines in part the
clinical course of unstable angina. The authors believe that this is the
first study in which inflammatory markers are compared with markers
of coagulation activity and endothelial function in a consecutive series
of patients with unstable angina. While the inflammatory markers —
namely, C-reactive protein, fibrinogen and sedimentation rate — may
only be a reflection of the underlying biological process triggered by
plaque rupture, a causal role cannot be excluded, and the inflammatory
markers may indeed indicate a proinflammatory state with consequent
negative effects on the healing process in the unstable plaque. Thus,
when plaque rupture occurs, the proinflammatory milieu may enhance
the process leading to persistent instability.

Largely unknown triggers may activate the endothelium to release
interleukin-6, which in turn stimulates the liver to produce C-reactive
protein. Some evidence suggests that CRP not only serves as a marker
in the acute phase response, but is also involved in pathogenesis. C-reactive protein may stimulate the production of tissue factor, the main
initiator of blood coagulation by mononuclear cells. CRP also reacts
with LDL and can activate the complement system. These properties
may contribute to plaque instability and influence the subsequent clinical course. The findings also suggest that fibrinogen, but not other hemostatic factors, is associated with prognosis and that fibrinogen may
influence the course of unstable angina in a way independent of its role
in hemostasis. In summary, the Leiden study supports the idea that increased inflammatory activity is a key mechanism in the pathophysiol-
ogy of unstable angina and a determinant of the clinical course. In the
population they studied — patients with severe unstable angina — a

proinflammatory state appears to be an important and independent determinant of short-term outcome.

In this same issue of the *European Heart Journal,* there is an editorial titled, "Inflammation and Outcome in Unstable Angina," by Curzen and Fox, that points out that the Leiden study found no association between inhospital outcome and markers of endothelial dysfunction. By contrast, in other situations involving vascular inflammatory responses, such as septic shock, the endothelium does play a pivotal role. The authors find it hard to conceive that a localized inflammatory response, as in severe unstable angina, would not affect and in turn be affected by the vascular endothelium.

Curzen and Fox suggest that an ultimate goal for patients admitted with unstable angina would be to have a blood test that would provide a somewhat reliable estimate of short-term risk as a guide to the necessity for cardiac catheterization and possible revascularization. While they concede that markers such as those studied in the Leiden paper as well as troponin-T and markers of endothelial function may contribute to prognosis, currently available data are not adequate to fully understand the significance of these parameters in risk stratification of patients with acute coronary syndromes.

In the *New England Journal of Medicine* for April 1997, Paul Ridker and his associates from Brigham and Women's Hospital, Harvard and the research laboratory at the University of Vermont, have a paper titled, "Inflammation, Aspirin and the Risk of Cardiovascular Disease in Apparently Healthy Men," in which they explore the role of inflammation in acute coronary syndromes. The authors found that baseline C-reactive protein levels did predict future risk of myocardial infarction and stroke. They also found that the degree of risk reduction caused by the use of aspirin after the first myocardial infarction appeared to be related directly to the level of C-reactive protein. The authors cite literature to show that inflammation has a role both in initiation and progression of the atherosclerotic process and that anti-inflammatory agents may have a role in the prevention of cardiovascular disease. They still believe, however, that data are not adequate to prove that inflammation increases the risk of first MI, stroke or venous thrombosis or that anti-inflammatory therapy per se reduces that risk.

The mechanism by which levels of C-reactive protein contribute to atherothrombosis is, of course, not clear. *Chlamydia pneumoniae, Helicobacter pylori,* herpes simplex and the cytomegaloviruses have been implicated as causes of chronic inflammation detected by CRP, which may be a surrogate for interleukin-6. C-reactive protein may also induce monocytes to express tissue factor, a membrane glycoprotein that is important in initiating coagulation.

The Ridker group's paper draws four major conclusions. The first is that C-reactive protein does predict risk of first MI and ischemic stroke independent of other factors. Second — and very interesting, I think — is that CRP is not associated with the risk of venous thrombosis, which is generally not associated with atherosclerosis. Third, C-reactive protein is not simply a short-term marker of risk, but also a long-term marker for events occurring years later. This in itself suggests that the effects of inflammation are part of a chronic process rather than an undetected acute illness. The final and very intriguing observation is that aspirin may be beneficial because of its anti-inflammatory properties as well as being an antiplatelet agent. The authors add the observation that C-reactive protein may be used to identify those patients more likely to be helped by aspirin.

Supporting the findings of the Verhaggen group's paper on the role of inflammatory factors in determining outcome in unstable angina is a 1994 paper in *Circulation* by van der Wal and associates from the University of Amsterdam titled, "Site of Intimal Rupture Erosion of Thrombosed Coronary Atherosclerotic Plaques as Characterized by Inflammatory Process Irrespective of the Dominant Plaque Morphology." The authors did an extensive post-mortem analysis on 20 patients who had acute myocardial infarction in which the site of plaque rupture of the implicated fatal coronary artery was traced in serial sections. They found that while the atherosclerotic plaque morphology was complicated and heterogeneous with respect to architecture and cellular composition, an inflammatory process was uniformly present. Their analysis suggests that inflammation had played a role in destabilizing the fibrous cap and thus enhancing the risk of the acute event.

In the *New England Journal* of August 1994, a paper by Attalio Maseri's group in Rome titled, "Prognostic Value of C-Reactive Protein and Serum Amyloid-A Protein in Unstable Angina," is important in the evolution of our understanding of the significance of CRP in acute coronary syndromes. In this study, C-reactive protein was measured in 31 patients with chronic unstable angina and 29 patients with acute myocardial infarction. At the time of admission, creatine kinase and troponin-T levels were normal, but CRP levels were elevated. The authors found that elevated C-reactive protein at the time of hospital admission did indeed reflect poor outcome in patients with unstable angina. Their results confirm and support a growing literature describing an inflammatory component in coronary disease.

38

Type II Diabetes, Coronary Artery Disease and Hypoglycemic Agents, Revisited

January 1999

In the journal *Heart* (formerly the *British Heart Journal*) there is an editorial whose title asks a question that at first glance may seem rather startling, but based on clinical and experimental data, it is actually quite reasonable and pertinent. The paper, "Diabetes and Coronary Artery Disease: Time to Stop Taking the Tablets?" is written by Connaughton and Webber from the Queen Elizabeth Hospital in Birmingham, England. It begins with the observation, not startling in itself, that patients with diabetes develop accelerated coronary artery disease and they are over-represented by 10 to 20 times among patients with acute myocardial infarction. The authors note that the mortality in diabetics with acute MI is twice that of non-diabetics and that coronary disease is the single most common cause of death among diabetic patients.

In spite of the wide prevalence of diabetes and the very high incidence of coronary disease among diabetics, the ideal treatment for diabetics with coronary disease is still not clear. In the United Kingdom, for example, there are about a million non-insulin-dependent diabetics who are more often than not treated with oral hypoglycemic agents, primarily the sulfonylureas. This is in spite of the fact that there has been a simmering controversy about oral hypoglycemic agents for some three decades, dating back to the University Group Diabetes Program Study, which suggested the possible role of oral hypoglycemic agents in the genesis of vascular complications in non-insulin-dependent diabetic patients. The authors cite Malmberg, writing in the *British Medical Journal* in 1997, who accumulated evidence for the superiority of insulin in treating diabetic patients following acute myocardial infarction.

Connaughton and Webber also cite animal studies in which the sulfonylureas caused coronary vasoconstriction with consequent myocardial ischemia. The hypoglycemic action of sulfonylureas is dependent on potassium adenosine triphosphate (ATP) channel closure, while the opening of potassium ATP channels in experimental animals has been shown to confer protection during myocardial ischemia. The authors note that there is evidence that potassium ATP channels may play an important role in the endogenous adaptation known as ischemic preconditioning. In addition, there are data showing that ischemic preconditioning may be blocked by sulfonylureas both in vitro and in vivo. The concentration of sulfonylureas required to do this is much higher than that required to produce pancreatic insulin release. Thus, it can be argued that these effects may not be pathophysiologically relevant. However, the sulfonylurea drugs may not only block preconditioning but may impede earlier responses to ischemia, such as coronary vasodilatation.

There is extensive literature on this subject. For example, in the January 1999 issue of the *Journal of the American College of Cardiology*, Garratt and colleagues from the Mayo Clinic have a paper entitled, "Sulfonylurea Drugs Increase Mortality in Patients with Diabetes Mellitus After Direct Angioplasty for Acute Myocardial Infarction." Their study concludes that this increased risk is not explained by ventricular arrhythmias, "but may reflect deleterious effects of sulfonylurea drugs on myocardial intolerance for ischemia and reperfusion." They add that in surviving patients, sulfonylurea drugs are not associated with increased late adverse events.

Garratt's group found that the risk of death for diabetic patients undergoing balloon angioplasty for acute MI is 2.7 times higher if they are using oral sulfonylurea hypoglycemic agents at the time of treatment. They also report that the impact of these drugs on early mortality is similar to that of low left ventricular ejection fraction or overt clinical heart failure. They suggest that the use of these drugs may represent an additional risk factor in patients undergoing interventional procedures in the presence of acute MI. The authors review supporting literature on this subject that includes references to increased cardiovascular mortality among type II diabetic patients taking oral agents and evidence that there was increased mortality of MI in diabetics treated with sulfonylureas compared to those treated with insulin. This increased mortality was not explained on the basis of age, differences in ventricular function, hypoglycemic control or procedural success.

Garrett and his co-authors also raise the possibility, based on experimental data, that the sulfonylureas may accelerate death of hypoxic cardiomyocytes through blockade of the potassium ATP channels. They cite evidence that these drugs abolish the cardioprotective effect of ischemic preconditioning in the isolated human myocardium and in patients undergoing balloon angioplasty. They also consider the question of whether sulfonylureas inhibit endogenous fibrinolysis.

In a 1996 issue of *Circulation*, Robert Engler of San Diego and Derrick Yellon of London contributed a paper entitled, "Sulfonylureas, Potassium ATP Blockade in Type II Diabetics and Preconditioning in Cardiovascular Disease: Time for Reconsideration." The authors believe that while there are no easy solutions, the fact that oral hypoglycemic agents inhibit the opening of the heart's endogenous protective potassium ATP channels should make us rethink the relative importance of this type of treatment. They point out that patients on such drugs tend to have larger myocardial infarctions. If preconditioning is clinically confirmed as a potent intervention, as it has been in the experimental laboratory, the therapeutic potential should be immense. In light of this, the authors pose the possibility that the use of sulfonylureas may block such potential therapeutic intervention.

Engler and Yellon observe that new discoveries often shed light on old mysteries and that this may be the case with the sulfonylurea class of oral hypoglycemic agents. For this reason, they believe, as do Connaughton and Webber, that it might be time to rethink the seeming paradoxical results of the 1970 University Group Diabetes Study. According to Engler and Yellon, non-insulin-dependent diabetic patients should be screened periodically for cardiovascular disease and risk factors and that sulfonylureas should perhaps be used only in patients who are at low risk. They propose a prospective trial of sulfonylureas in diabetics that includes screening for cardiovascular disease since the original University Group Diabetes Program Study enrolled all type II patients, not just those with cardiovascular disease. The bottom line for Engler and Yellon is that there should be more cautious use of sulfonylureas in patients at risk for cardiovascular disease.

In a 1997 issue of *Circulation*, there is an article by Cleveland and associates from the University of Colorado entitled, "Oral Sulfonylurea Hypoglycemic Agents Prevent Ischemic Preconditioning in the Human Myocardium: Two Paradoxes Revisited." Their data suggest that the long-term use of oral hypoglycemic agents blocks the protection given by ischemic preconditioning and that long-term inhibition of potassium ATP channels with oral agents may explain the excess cardiovascular mortality in the patients taking these agents. The authors consider biguanide agents as an alternative to the sulfonylureas. While these drugs don't have the adverse effects on the potassium ATP channels, they may cause other problems, such as lactic acidosis, for which intravascular radiographic contrast media may need to be used.

In their editorial, Connaughton and Webber conclude that if insulin was shown to have a clear advantage over oral hypoglycemic agents in type II diabetics, it would have a major impact on public health with all the associated problems caused by wholesale conversion to insulin, including patient acceptance and monitoring costs, among many other factors. They recognize that clinical trials to answer these questions will require sufficient statistical power to detect what might be rather small absolute differences in outcome, with some parallels to the thrombolytic studies that have made such an important contribution with their mega-trials.

Based on current theoretical and clinical evidence, Connaughton and Webber believe that diabetics should be treated with insulin during the acute phase of myocardial infarction and that this treatment should be continued indefinitely thereafter. They add, more speculatively, that sulfonylureas should not be given to diabetic patients with coronary disease. They also suggest that some mention of the potential for antagonism between potassium channel openers and sulfonylureas should be added to the British National Formulary. Engler and Yellon note in their paper that the package inserts for all sulfonylurea drugs do carry a warning of possible increased cardiovascular mortality. All this notwithstanding, Connaughton and Webber concede that the time has not yet come to stop all use of oral hypoglycemics because the clinical evidence does not support the superiority of insulin in type II diabetic patients with coronary disease. But they do believe that it is time to implement trials that are capable of answering these important questions that have such enormous economic and medical public health implications.

I find this series of articles to be compelling, provocative and illustrative of how important it is to challenge conventional medical thinking and practices that all too often tend to become ingrained, sometimes for years. While this discussion may not have produced any answers, at least it raises some important clinical and intellectual questions that will need to be answered.

39

Treatment of Hypertension: A Metaphor for Medicine — Advanced Looking Backward, Primitive Looking Forward

January 1998

1 997 was the 25th anniversary of the National High Blood Pressure Education Program established in 1972 by the National Heart, Lung and Blood Institute. The first report of the Joint National Committee on Detection, Evaluation and Treatment of High Blood Pressure came out in 1977 and once every four years thereafter. The most recent one, JNC 6, was released several weeks ago.

In commemoration of the 25th anniversary of the National High Blood Pressure Education Program, Dr. Marvin Moser has written a delightful and perceptive monograph titled, "Myths, Misconceptions and Heroics: The Story of the Treatment of Hypertension from the 1930s." Moser begins his monograph with a quotation from *The Life of Galileo* by Bertold Brecht: "The aim of science is not to open a door to endless wisdom, but to put a limit to endless error." The latter part of this quote, I believe, is especially applicable to the history of hypertensive treatment.

In 1931, Dr. Paul Dudley White observed, "Hypertension may be an important compensatory mechanism which should not be tampered with, even were it certain that we could control it." In the same year, in the *British Medical Journal*, one Dr. Hay, a distinguished British physician of the time, said something similar: "The greatest danger to a man with high blood pressure lies in its discovery, because then some fool is certain to try to reduce it." These views were probably appropriate at that time, considering the methods of treatment that were then available. It was also believed at the time that hypertension was an essential adaptive mechanism, perhaps leading to the term "essential hypertension." This idea was expressed by Scott in the 1947 edition of *Tice's Practice of Medicine*, when he asked, "May not the elevation of systemic blood pressure be a natural response to guarantee a more normal circulation to the heart and kidneys?"

Moser points out that in the 1920s and 1930s, restriction of fat and cholesterol intake was advocated, but for the wrong reasons. At that time, it was thought that a high-protein diet might contribute to kidney disease, which was then thought to be the principal cause of high blood pressure. While it was known that a high salt intake was associated with high blood pressure and stroke, most cases of high blood pressure went largely untreated for want of even minimally effective medicines. A good example of this is the case of President Franklin Delano Roosevelt. In 1935, at the age of 53, his blood pressure was 136/78. In 1940, when he was elected to his third term as President, it was between 170/90 and 180/100. The treatment he received was phenobarbital, a low-salt, low-fat diet and massages. Later, Roosevelt's blood pressure reached a level of 180/105, his heart was enlarged and in all probability, he had already suffered lacunar infarcts. By 1944, his blood pressure was as high as 230/126, and congestive heart failure and renal failure had supervened. FDR died from cerebral vascular hemorrhage in 1945, when he was 63. Moser cites Roosevelt's history as typical of the desperate state of high blood pressure treatment in the 1930s and 1940s.

The 1940s and 1950s saw the use of the Kempner diet which advocated fruits, vegetables, rice and more rice — a diet limited to 20 grams of protein, 5 grams of fat and less than 200 milligrams of sodium per day. In some cases, this diet did cause improvement, but it was brutal and difficult to follow. Sir George Pickering, the great British physician-philosopher, described the Kempner diet as "insipid, unappetizing, monotonous, unacceptable and intolerable," requiring "the asceticism of a religious zealot." Perhaps the same might be said of some diets that are advocated today in the management of coronary disease.

This was also the era of surgical sympathectomy, which, even though it might temporarily have halted the progression of severe hypertension in perhaps 40 to 50 percent of patients, came at a high price. Not only did it require hospitalization for as long as six to eight weeks, but it often caused severe postural hypotension, syncope and impotence. Intravenous sodium amytol was given preoperatively, and if the blood pressure didn't decrease, the disease was considered too severe even for surgery. In spite of the difficulties, surgical sympathectomy did lay the groundwork for the development of medications for sympathetic blockade to reduce high blood pressure.

Moser's monograph recalls the various medications prescribed for high blood pressure over the years. In the 1930s, veratrum alkaloids and phenobarbital were used. In the 1940s, Drs. Ed Freis and Irvine Page began vasodilator treatment, and for the first time, there was some resolution of malignant hypertension. Thiocyanates, ganglion blocking agents and Rauwolfia derivatives were also sometimes prescribed during this time. In the 1950s, guanethidine and monoamine oxidase inhibitors appeared along with hydralazine, which is still in use today. Effective diuretics also date from the late 1950s. In the 1960s came beta blockers, and in the 1970s, angiotensin-converting enzyme inhibitors. Calcium channel blockers appeared in the 1980s, and angiotensin II antagonists in the 1990s.

In 1955, Perrara estimated that the life expectancy of a hypertensive patient was 52 years. The untreated condition appeared to run a course of about 20 years, with little or no symptoms for 10 years and then complications becoming frequent, including congestive heart failure, renal failure and stroke. By the 1990s, the onset of congestive heart failure in treated hypertensives was long delayed in comparison to the patient treated for high blood pressure in the 1950s. As longevity in hypertensive patients increased, a great many cases of congestive heart failure appeared, but they occurred much later in life. This effect has caused a major challenge to our current practice and is a grim reminder that today, even our most effective treatments delay rather than prevent the inevitable.

In 1966, in his famous textbook, *Diseases of the Heart* — one of the last written by a single author — Charles Friedberg said that in a patient with mild, benign hypertension — that is, with a blood pressure less than 220/100 — there was no indication for the use of hypotensive drugs. Rather, he believed that careful observation and conservative treatment consisting of reassurance, mild sedatives and weight reduction were desirable. As late as 1974, a *Lancet* paper concluded that antihypertensive agents produced no obvious benefit in patients over 65 years of age, and in 1978, an editorial in the *British Medical Journal* advised that hypotensive drugs should probably not be used in elderly patients unless their blood pressure was more than 200/110.

Beginning in the 1960s and flourishing by the 1980s, major clinical trials began to establish that the early treatment of high blood pressure would indeed prevent and delay complications and prolong life. In the first Joint National Committee report of 1977, the "step therapy" was advocated, a treatment that began with diuretics and reserpine, then propranolol as the second step and hydralazine as the third. This approach generated its own set of controversies and as time passed and as medications changed, one rarely hears the term "step therapy" any more.

Even a cursory review of some of the ACCEL interviews of the early 1970s highlights the monumental progress that has occurred in the management of hypertension since that time. For example, Dr. Ed Fries, a leading hypertension specialist of the time, was asked, What evidence is there that antihypertensive drugs prevent morbidity and mortality? His answer alluded to the favorable effects of medication on signs and symptoms of malignant hypertension, a diagnosis rarely made today. Fries cited then-recent evidence that antihypertensive drugs prevented complications in patients with diastolic blood pressures of 115 to 130, which he said were below the pressures of patients with malignant hypertension.

It is humbling for a doctor practicing today to realize how many of the treatments once embraced so enthusiastically and thought to be harbingers of future success have become merely footnotes in the history of medicine. This is illustrated in a discussion on ACCEL between Dr. Al Soffer of Chicago, at the time editor of *Chest*, and Dr. Al Brest of the University of Pennsylvania, a distinguished expert in hypertension, who expressed enthusiasm for the potential of carotid sinus nerve stimulation in the treatment of high blood pressure.

In reviewing the past efforts of doctors to treat malignant hypertension and renal failure with the limited medications available to them, it is no wonder that Marvin Moser quotes Al Sjoerdsma, who wrote in *Circulation* in 1963: "I look on the work of physicians who pursued the drug approach in hypertension as being well nigh heroic." It may not be too long before future cardiologists and cardiovascular surgeons will look back at the many interventions that we prize so highly today — catheters, stents, heart/lung machines and a myriad of other devices — and marvel at how we carried on so boldly and so proudly with what may then seem like primitive technologies.

40

A Spectrum of Clinical Judgments: A Patient with Stroke and Unstable Angina

July 1995

W e practice at a time when all medical decisions are being closely scrutinized by non-medical organizations such as insurance companies, HMOs and various managed care hybrids. Frequently, they require permission to hospitalize patients and then permission to proceed with diagnostic and surgical interventions. At times, reimbursement is disallowed retrospectively by agents for third-party organizations who are far removed from the clinical scene. Underlying these policies is the assumption that every medical condition can be readily codified and that there is a right and wrong approach that can be defined by protocol.

In the *British Medical Journal* for June 3, 1995, there is a case presentation that illustrates the complexity and difficulty of making medical decisions, and perhaps even more important, it shows how expert and sophisticated doctors often disagree in their clinical judgment. The article, "How Should a Patient Presenting with Unstable Angina and a Recent Stroke be Managed?" is written by investigators from the University Department of Clinical Neurosciences at Western General Hospital in Edinburgh. A 60-year-old, right-handed bartender with a 12-month history of exertional chest pain and more recently, chest pain at rest, was referred for possible coronary angiography. An electrocardiogram showed a Q-wave interior wall myocardial infarction. There was a moderately positive exercise stress test. Previous treatment had included atenolol, nitrates and aspirin. The day before referral, right arm and leg weakness occurred, with partial, nominal aphasia. Symptoms waxed and waned. Motor function varied from a loss of fine finger movement in the right hand to complete right-arm paralysis. The right leg was affected to a lesser degree. Coronary arteriography was deferred and the patient was transferred to the neurological service. A

CT scan (computed tomography) showed an old, right cerebellar infarct and nothing more. Carotid ultrasound suggested right internal carotid occlusion and 90+ percent stenosis of the left carotid. Neurological symptoms continued to fluctuate.

Immediate diagnostic and therapeutic options were discussed by cardiologists, neurologists and vascular surgeons from the United States and Britain. John Porter, Professor of Surgery at the Oregon Health Sciences University in Portland, favored left carotid endarterectomy without delay. He suggested that in this situation — fluctuating neurological symptoms with high-grade carotid stenosis — CT scans are notoriously unreliable in defining stroke and therefore, he required an MRI. If there was no evidence of stroke, Dr. Porter said he would proceed with carotid endarterectomy without angiography to investigate the coronary artery status. If there was a non-hemorrhagic stroke, he would maintain the patient on heparin for several days prior to endarterectomy, based on what he called his unproved impression that this treatment often decreased postoperative morbidity. It's important that this consultant based his judgment on what he considered an unproved impression. I mention this only to suggest that this is an entirely defensible position and that it is not possible for every decision in medicine to be based on incontrovertible or proven data. Dr. Porter conceded that this patient would be at increased risk of perioperative myocardial infarction, but, although others might disagree, he felt that a combined coronary-carotid procedure had a substantially higher risk of morbidity and mortality than either procedure done separately. He opposed subjecting this neurologically unstable patient to coronary angiography and a possible combined procedure, and instead favored immediate carotid revascularization.

Drs. Philip Hornick and K.M. Taylor of the Department of Cardiothoracic Surgery at the Hammersmith Hospital in London thought that in this case, carotid endarterectomy and coronary bypass surgery should be performed as a single procedure. They believed that the pooled data show that the risk of stroke is about the same for staged and combined procedures, but that there is a higher incidence of myocardial infarction and a higher mortality for staged procedures.

Magnus Ohman, Assistant Professor of Medicine at Duke, believed that the most unstable vascular condition should be treated first and that this could be decided only by carotid and cardiac angiography. He made what I think is a wise observation that while randomized trials may define the best approach to patients with unstable angina and multivessel coronary disease or symptomatic carotid disease, the benefit-to-risk ratio of carotid endarterectomy, coronary bypass grafting or a combined procedure in patients with both carotid and coronary disease can be assessed only retrospectively. Ohman believed that combined carotid and coronary procedures should be reserved for patients with high-risk unstable angina, severe left ventricular dysfunction and left main disease or its equivalent, in which case perioperative hypotension or ischemia during the carotid endarterectomy could become irreversible. Believing that in this case the coronary disease placed the patient only at intermediate cardiological risk, but at high neurological risk, he favored carotid endarterectomy as an isolated procedure.

Graham Jackson, a consultant at Guy's Hospital in London, thought that this patient needed carotid surgery by an experienced vascular surgeon. He explored various options and concluded that if stable angina were present, carotid surgery should be done and, if needed, it should be followed in a few days with bypass surgery. If the angina were unstable, he would favor a combined procedure.

Now for the real-life results. The patient did have both carotid and coronary angiography. There was a 95 percent stenosis of the left carotid artery. The right carotid artery was occluded. Cardiac catheterization showed left ventricular impairment with triple vessel disease. The patient had carotid endarterectomy based on the decision that the coronary disease was stable and that myocardial revascularization could be delayed. Carotid surgery was successful. The patient was discharged with only mild impairment of fine finger movement of the right hand. Coronary bypass surgery would be done in due course.

Thus the opinions for treatment for this patient varied from immediate carotid surgery without coronary artery investigation, to coronary and carotid angiography, and based on the findings, a possible combined procedure. Is there a right and wrong approach in this kind of complex situation? Can anyone sit in judgment and purport to authorize or deny one approach or the other, prospectively or retrospectively? The success of any of these approaches requires consummate medical science. But the judgment as to how to apply that science is still an art, and perhaps an art that is not possible to define or quantify. Not to be forgotten are the intangibles and the variations from patient to patient in what may seem retrospectively to be similar situations. These intangibles may well affect the result in an entirely unpredictable way. While giving a great deal of medical information, this case presentation does not discuss the individual patient, the family or personal considerations that may also play an important role in decision-making.

As David Blumenthal of Harvard points out in his commentary in the spring 1994 edition of *Health Affairs*, no amount of external quality monitoring or regulatory intervention will fully correct what economists so delicately call the "asymmetries of information" that exist between doctors and patients in a given situation. In his discussion of the vital importance of maintaining professionalism in healthcare reform, Blumenthal states that in their hour of need, patients rely on the knowledge of the physician to protect and maximize their health. He goes on to say that in most clinical situations, the medical knowledge base is sufficient to dictate proper treatment and that guidelines and protocols, while a starting point for development of practice standards, are not an end in themselves.

The patient from Edinburgh illustrates the wide latitude inherent in the exercise of medical judgment. In his discussion of the dangers to medical professionalism in the current healthcare environment, Blumenthal emphasizes that federal and state authorities — and I would add as even more pertinent, the commercial institutions that control a good bit of medicine — should be careful "to avoid the reality or appearance of removing the power of professionals through counterproductive efforts to limit professional autonomy." And he adds, "this is a particular danger where guidelines are concerned."

But how to provide a milieu for proper diagnosis and treatment in an increasingly stylized and regulated system, especially for patients with complicated medical problems, will remain, I fear, a conundrum far more difficult to solve than the case from Edinburgh.

41

Myocardial Revascularization: A Time of Change and Controversy

March 1999

The March 1999 scientific sessions of the American College of Cardiology, held this year in New Orleans, were, in my opinion, among the most exciting in recent years, reflecting a literal ferment of research and innovation in virtually every phase of cardiology. Nowhere are these changes more evident than in the field of myocardial revascularization. Controversy and change now abound in bypass surgery, which for many years was a stable, if not static, widely used and highly successful approach to myocardial revascularization. But now, what we euphemistically call minimally invasive and off-pump procedures are challenging both conventional bypass surgery and catheter-based techniques, which themselves are in constant evolution. And not to be overlooked is laser epicardial transmyocardial surgical revascularization, with endocardial catheter-based techniques looming as an alternative, even while epicardial revascularization strives for validation and acceptance. If that were not enough, there are totally new and different methods of revascularization in progress, some of which are reflected in the papers presented in New Orleans, including cellular cardioplasty, the pathology of angiogenesis and various genetic interventions to achieve angiogenesis.

While changing concepts in medicine and surgery are never lacking for fervent advocates and naysayers, there is especially sharp division on the issue of minimally invasive bypass surgery. In a recent article in *Circulation* entitled, "Minimally Invasive Coronary Bypass: A Dissenting Opinion," Larry Bonchek and Dan Ullyot, both distinguished cardiac surgeons, present a critique for the purpose of stimulating discussion and debate. Bonchek and Ullyot concede at the outset that it's difficult to argue against attempts to minimize the invasiveness of any procedure, but they believe that procedures such as arthroscopy and laparoscopic cholecystectomy that involve a minimum of precision

— almost no sewing, as they put it — cannot be compared to the physiologically and technically complex cardiac operations.

The authors point to 30 years of successful bypass surgery, which they describe as "safe, effective, durable, reproducible, complete, versatile and teachable." In their view, the success of bypass surgery depends on several critical components, including uncompromising selection of optimal sites for microvascular anastomoses, ability to manage unexpected circumstances, and not least of all, complete multivessel revascularization. They defend the median sternotomy incision and its adequate exposure as a basic ingredient of all good cardiac surgery. Advocates of non-pump, beating-heart and minimally invasive direct coronary artery bypass (MIDCAB) surgery claim that the incisions are better tolerated, cosmetically more acceptable and less apt to cause morbidity than cardiopulmonary bypass. With regard to port-access, on-pump surgery, incisional morbidity is said to be less, recovery faster, and costs are reduced because of shorter hospital stays.

Bonchek and Ullyot contend, however, that operations using these small incisions are actually longer and technically more difficult than standard bypass. Applicability may be limited by peripheral vascular disease, aortic regurgitation and ischemic mitral regurgitation. While MIDCAB surgery for left internal mammary artery (LIMA) to left anterior descending artery (LAD) for proximal disease may divert some patients from percutaneous transluminal coronary angioplasty (PTCA) and stent, Bonchek and Ullyot fear that surgeons will begin to do the very thing for which they have criticized cardiologists — fail to produce complete revascularization. They point to frequent MIDCAB anastomotic failures and the extensive learning curve for which vulnerable patients may pay a high price.

Bonchek and Ullyot believe that the demand for such procedures is created by promotional advertising that is aimed at a poorly informed and gullible public who are led to believe that these techniques are widely applicable and that the results are comparable to standard bypass surgery. They also suggest that these misconceptions are further encouraged by equipment manufacturers. Their view can perhaps best be epitomized by a direct quote: "Minimally invasive coronary bypass seductively promises short-term benefits with no proof as yet that it can match the long-term benefits of the standard operation which are firmly established and thoroughly documented." Finally, Bonchek and Ullyot say that advocates of these new surgical procedures are shifting onto others the burden of proving that they are not only beneficial, but can be performed by any competent surgeon without compromising safety and durability. They say they're waiting for such evidence.

In the March 23, 1999 issue of *Circulation*, there are two editorials that prove that the Bonchek-Ullyot editorial has indeed achieved its stated goal of stimulating discussion and debate on the issue of minimally invasive surgery. The first editorial, by Cornelius Borst and Paul Grundeman from Utrecht in the Netherlands, is titled, "Minimally Invasive Coronary Artery Bypass Grafting: An Experimental Perspective." In this editorial, the authors present an opinion opposite to that of Bonchek and Ullyot. They challenge the assertion that standard bypass procedures are "safe, effective, durable, reproducible, complete, versatile and teachable." They point to the Society of Thoracic Surgeons (STS) national cardiac surgical database (January 1998), which cites an operative mortality of 2.9 percent (2.5 percent for men and 0.4 percent for women) with the mortality increasing from 1.1 percent for ages 20 to 50 to 7.2 percent for ages 81 to 90. It also indicates that 65 percent of procedures have no complications. Borst and Grundeman accept that there are solid reasons for performing coronary bypass surgery on an arrested heart — it is empty, flaccid and can be manipulated easily to expose all branches — but they believe that these advantages do not come easily for patients, particularly if they are elderly.

In conventional bypass surgery, there are often subtle postoperative changes from microthrombi due to platelet activation and gaseous emboli as well as a systemic inflammatory process induced by extracorporeal circulation manifested by fever, activation of leukocytes, C-reactive protein and a host of other factors. There also are arrhythmias, endothelial dysfunction, interstitial fluid accumulation and pulmonary and renal dysfunction. It is these elements of morbidity and mortality attributable to conventional bypass surgery that invite exploration for techniques that have fewer adverse effects. Borst and Grundeman believe that in five years, 50 percent of coronary bypass surgery will be performed on a beating heart mainly with arterial conduits through a closed chest, and that one ought not to be deterred from searching for new methods if so much is to be gained for so many patients.

The second editorial in *Circulation* that responds to the Bonchek-Ullyot editorial is called, "Inertia of Success" and it is co-authored by Michael Mack of Dallas; Ralph Damiano of Hershey, Pennsylvania; Robert Matheny of Indianapolis; Herman Reichenspurg of Munich and Alain Carpentier of Paris. They begin with a quotation from Henri Bergson: "To exist is to change, to change is to mature, to mature is to go on recreating oneself endlessly." With this quotation they position themselves philosophically on the high ground in the search for progress, facing whatever perils and risks there may be, rather than defending the status quo, which they perceive as less than perfect. While they agree with Bonchek and Ullyot that unbridled enthusiasm and a blind eye toward critical analysis are dangerous, in their opinion, it is equally precarious to think that we have an operation that cannot or should not be made better. They say that "we are at a strategic inflection point in surgery and are in danger of becoming obsolete." They very effectively use the analogy of the typewriter, which made valuable contributions to information systems in the past, but which now has been made obsolete by the computer.

Mack and his co-authors further contest Bonchek and Ullyot on some aspects of the isolated left internal mammary to left anterior descending procedure. According to the STS database, this operation comprises only 2 percent of bypass procedures. If this operation is as safe, simple, rapid and successful as Bonchek and Ullyot say, why are people opting for the less invasive LAD revascularization by catheter techniques? They also question Bonchek and Ullyot on the issue of incomplete revascularization. They ask whether every octogenarian, for example, with a critical proximal LAD lesion and a chronically occluded right coronary artery with good collateralization requires a median sternotomy to add a second graft to the right coronary artery. In other words, they contend that there are instances where, on balance, less than complete revascularization may be appropriate. Mack and his co-authors go on to say that while it may be true that some patients following traditional bypass are dismissed in three to four days, most are not. The STS database describes a 6.6-day average stay for patients having first-time elective operations, and they ask how many of these patients leave the hospital after three to four days with the functional capacity for work or recreation in one or two weeks, which is often the case after minimally invasive surgery. Mack and his colleagues also resent the implication that minimally invasive operations are aggressively marketed to a gullible public. They say that beating-heart surgery is pursued because of its many advantages, including that of avoiding the sequellae of cardiopulmonary bypass, but they concede that the procedure cannot yet be compared with the long-term benefits of conventional surgery because it has only been performed for three years.

In answer to Bonchek and Ullyot's claim that the burden of proof of the effectiveness of minimally invasive surgery should be on those who propose it, Mack and his co-authors cite some eight papers in which the results are comparable, at least up to this point, to any published series on graft patency by conventional bypass surgery. They further state that MIDCAB surgery is the most closely scrutinized operation ever at this early stage of its evolution. Regarding the argument that only a few virtuosos can perform the operation, they point out that 20 years ago, the mitral valve repair could only be done by a few master surgeons and now it is performed effectively by many surgeons. In fairness, however, some might question whether valve repair is really comparable to standard open heart bypass techniques.

In summary, Mack and his co-authors believe that notwithstanding the great good done by traditional bypass surgery during the past 30 years, the treatment can still be improved. They are intrigued by the so-called hybrid or integrated coronary revascularizations that combine the superior outcome of LIMA to LAD using the MIDCAB technique with less invasive catheter techniques for other vessels. While these three editorials can perhaps be described in gentlest terms as confrontational, they are indicative of the sea change now inevitable in the field of bypass surgery — and it is more change than we would ever have imagined only a few years ago. Beyond that, as the Mack editorial suggests, the issue of standard bypass surgery versus minimally invasive surgery is by no means the only frontier in the field of myocardial revascularization today.

Laser transmyocardial revascularization, genetic stimulation and other ways of promoting angiogenesis may in time render this debate on traditional bypass surgery versus minimally invasive techniques, if not obsolete, at least far less important than it now appears. Great strides in the prevention of atherothrombosis and methods of revascularization that are more attractive and far less invasive than any form of surgery we know of today, may not be as far off as we may now think.

42

The Twilight of Coronary Disease?

May 1996

T
he May 3, 1996 issue of *Science* focuses on cardiovascular medicine in a section called, "Frontiers in Biomedicine." It is keynoted by an optimistic and provocative editorial by Nobel Laureates Michael Brown and Joseph Goldstein. Entitled, "Heart Attacks: Gone with This Century?" the editorial takes a look at the role of genes in controlling the formation of the heart and their contribution to the development of high blood pressure and inherited arrhythmias and cardiomyopathies.

One of the articles in this section, by Breslow from Rockefeller University, describes a mouse model of atherosclerosis. Although mice are highly resistant to atherosclerosis, genetic mutations can produce a strain that is deficient in apolipoprotein E with arteriosclerotic lesions that are similar to those observed in humans. These lesions are exaggerated by high-cholesterol, high-fat, Western-type diets. Mice and other mutants that that are deficient in LDL receptors, can be used to study the pathogenesis of atherosclerotic lesions and the influence of environment, hormones and drugs.

An article by Gary Gibbons and Victor Dzau of Stanford considers molecular therapies for vascular disease. To put it briefly, atherosclerosis is the most common form of occlusive vascular disease. The authors suggest that the pathogenesis of atherosclerosis involves a series of critical events, including endothelial dysfunction, infiltration of inflammatory cells into the vessel wall, alterations in vascular cell phenotype and vascular remodeling. The ability to reduce risk factors such as elevated cholesterol and interventions such as balloon angioplasty and bypass surgery will become more effective as the molecular basis for pathogenetic events is better understood. Gibbons and Dzau point to restenosis as a paradigm for molecular therapy and cite several molecular therapies that have already been designed and tested on animal models, one of which may be the replacement of nitric oxide synthase, a key product of endothelial cells. Others may include cytotoxic therapy and local radiation to inhibit neointimal formation after vascular injury.

With regard to vein bypass graft failure, the authors mention genetically engineered grafts that are resistant to atherosclerosis when implanted in rabbits with severe hyperlipidemia. This is just one example of the future possibility of applying genetic engineering technology to vascular bypass graft surgery. Vascular grafts may be used in the future as carrier systems for implanting cells that are genetically engineered. Gibbons and Dzau emphasize the necessity of finding an effective animal experimental model that can be used to predict the effects of various medications in humans, a problem that continues to be most vexing. They also question whether extensive clinical trials to demonstrate reduction in clinical events — for example, myocardial infarction and mortality — are really prerequisites for the approval of new vascular therapeutic agents.

In their editorial, Brown and Goldstein present the sanguine view that heart attacks, recognized as a public health issue only in this century, may "lose this notoriety" in the next century — a prediction that is based on four decades of progress in understanding cholesterol and lipoproteins that carry it in blood plasma. They cite the following research results that define the role of LDL in atherogenesis. First, they cite experimental results in which animals with low levels of LDL have no atherosclerosis and manipulations that raise LDL universally cause the disease. Second, they give the epidemiological evidence that human populations with low LDL levels have little atherosclerosis and the disease increases in all populations as LDL levels rise. And third, they cite the evidence that genetic mutations that impair receptor-mediated removal of LDL cause explosive atherosclerosis.

Brown and Goldstein emphasize three major studies, all of which were completed during the last 18 months, that show the effectiveness of statins in inhibiting CoA reductase, a key enzyme of cholesterol synthesis. These studies are the Scandinavian Simvastatin Survival Study (4S study) and two more recently reported studies, the West of Scotland Study (WOSCOPS) and one from North America, the Cholesterol and Recurrent Events study (CARE). The authors believe that these studies, which used statins to reduce LDL levels by 26 to 35 percent, would have been even more effective had cholesterol been lowered further and earlier. Conceding that while the therapeutic trials tell us that atherosclerosis can be reduced by lowering LDL with statins, the authors ask, are these trials safe? Three recent statin trials that were conducted over a five-year period with 7500 patients showed no significant increase in noncardiac deaths. While acknowledging that these studies are reassuring, they also think they are brief and that long-term studies are needed. They wonder whether hidden toxicity will emerge after individuals take these drugs for most of their lives. Nevertheless, the authors believe that in middle-aged people with cholesterol levels greater than 240, the potential for coronary disease warrants aggressive cholesterol lowering by diet and drugs. Brown and Goldstein warn that if we wait for susceptible individuals to develop symptoms before we treat them, the earliest symptom may be sudden death.

Now, perhaps as a counterpoint, I will call your attention to some letters to the editor of the *New England Journal of Medicine* that appeared in the May 16, 1996 issue. Stewart Rogers of Greensboro, North Carolina, in a letter discussing the West of Scotland Study, points out that the net benefit of taking pravastatin (40 mg a day for five years as compared to placebo) was a 2.2 percent reduction in the combined endpoints of nonfatal myocardial infarction and death from coronary disease, or a 0.7 percent reduction in the incidence of death from cardiovascular disease. This would mean that 45 men with hypercholesterolemia must be treated for five years to prevent one combined endpoint and 143 must be treated to prevent one death from a cardiac cause. Based on current costs of pravastatin, this would mean $6000 a year or $270,000 worth of pravastatin would be needed to prevent one combined endpoint, and more than $850,000 to prevent one death from a cardiac cause. For women, the projected cost to prevent one death would be $3.4 million.

In a letter regarding the 4S study and the West of Scotland Study, Drs. Samani and DeBono of the University of Leicester in England, state that the West of Scotland Study does give unequivocal evidence that primary treatment of moderate hypercholesterolemia is effective and it supports the results of the 4S study, but they ask how the results of these two landmark studies should be incorporated into clinical practice. They make the observation that the 4S study shows that the absolute benefits of treatment are approximately three to six times higher in the setting of secondary prevention. They point out that in the 4S study, the probability of survival over the six-year period is 87.7 percent and that with treatment, it is increased only, as they put it, to 91.3 percent using simvastatin. In the West of Scotland Study, survival over a period of five years is increased from 96 to 97 percent. Even though these results are most likely cumulative, Samani and DeBono wonder how many asymptomatic patients will be prepared to take lifelong medication for this sort of gain.

Dr. Stewart Cobbe and the other authors of the West of Scotland

Study answer that mortality is not the only valid endpoint, especially in a study on primary prevention, and that the reduction in morbidity shown quite clearly in the West of Scotland Study is also of key importance. Answering a further question regarding the use of simvastatin in older age groups, Dr. Peterson of the 4S study points out that toward the end of the study, when patients were between 70 and 75 years of age, the difference between the placebo and simvastatin groups was at its very highest. Thus, he believes that in the upper age groups, treatment may yet be effective.

Brown and Goldstein — who feel we must develop noninvasive screening methods capable of detecting coronary atherosclerosis in its earlier stages — close their editorial with the thought that the proof of the cholesterol hypothesis, the discovery of effective drugs and the improved definition of genetic susceptibility factors may well put an end to coronary disease as a major public health problem in the next century. While many may consider this an extravagant assessment of present prospects, it comes from two authorities with impeccable credentials in this field. Perhaps our challenge, whether as clinicians or as researchers, is to use the tools we have at hand to their best advantage to make the prediction of Brown and Goldstein come true.

43

Heart Rate and Longevity: Their Relationship and Clinical Implications

October 1997

In the *Journal of the American College of Cardiology* for October 1997, there is an intriguing editorial by Herbert J. Levine from the Tufts Medical School and the New England Medical Center in Boston. Unlike most of what we talk about on ACCEL, Levine's editorial has nothing to do with diagnosis, treatment, healthcare reform or a new randomized clinical trial. Yet his paper, "Resting Heart Rate and Life Expectancy," commands attention with its haunting suggestion that life span may be predetermined by the basic energetics of living cells, that perhaps there is an inverse relationship between life span and heart rate, and the possibility that each species has a predetermined number of heart beats in its lifetime.

Levine first points out that smaller mammals have higher heart rates and shorter life spans than larger ones. He describes a biophysical imperative that the ratio of heat loss (a function of body surface area) to heat production (a function of body mass) increases as body size is reduced. A mathematical analysis of body weight and metabolic rate of mammals yields a straight line, with exactly the same slope as a plot between body mass and heart rate. In all mammals, except for humans, there is a linear, inverse, semilogarithmic relationship between heart rate and life expectancy that spans a 35-fold difference in heart rate and a 20-fold difference in life span. Levine speculates that the life span of humans is different partially because science, medicine and sociological factors have allowed modern humans to stretch the boundaries of biology to permit a life expectancy of 80 years.

Plotting heart beats per lifetime against life expectancy in mammals shows that even for a 40-fold difference in life expectancy, the number of heart beats per lifetime, in order of magnitude, is remarkably constant. The total number of heart beats per lifetime in mammals, plotted against body mass, is also strikingly constant. This seems even more impressive if one considers that in mammals as small as the hamster up to those as large as the whale, this relationship is constant over a span of half a million-fold in body weight. In large and small mammals, the relationship of heart weight to body weight is almost linear, with heart weights remaining constant in a range of 0.05 to 0.06 percent of body weight. The same relationship exists between heart weight and heart beats per lifetime in mammals. Even though this relationship has not been analyzed in non-mammalian vertebrates, there is reason to believe that it is valid. A Galapagos tortoise, for example, whose life expectancy is 177 years, has a heart rate of six beats per minute.

According to Levine, the possibility cannot be excluded that resting heart rate may prove to be a determinant of life span. He asks the still unanswerable question of whether there may be a potential to prolong life by reducing average heart rate. In Levine's words: "If humans are predetermined to have in the neighborhood of three billion heart beats in a lifetime, would a reduction in the average rate extend life? And if so, one might estimate that the reduction in mean heart rate from 70 to 60 beats throughout life might increase the life span from 80 to more than 90 years."

This experiment, of course, has never been performed in humans, but Levine cites the study of Coburn and associates that appeared in the *Johns Hopkins Medical Journal* in 1971, in which digoxin — admittedly in doses that would be fatal for humans — increased survival in mice whose heart rates had been slowed. The study's data were confounded, however, by a lower body weight in the digoxin-treated mice, although they had a caloric intake comparable to the control mice. Even so, the role of cardiac slowing in the prolongation of life in digoxin-treated mice remains, at best, uncertain. A reduction in myocardial metabolic rate, with an associated reduction in heart rate, might have the potential to extend human life, but because myocardial oxygen consumption per unit weight is the same in normal, hypertrophied and failing hearts, the demonstration that a primary reduction in heart rate prolongs life would have to invoke a mechanism other than reduction in metabolic rate. In spite of this problem, Levine refers to clinical studies suggesting that heart rate slowing may improve survival, giving the obvious example of beta blockade following myocardial infarction. He further suggests that cardiac slowing may help patients with dilated cardiomyopathy and also cites the bradycardic effects of regular exercise. However, whether or not this slowing of the heart is a specific factor in improving longevity is not known.

In a paper in the *Journal of the American College of Cardiology* in 1992, Frits Meijler and his colleagues compare mammals with regard to heart size, AV conduction and heart rate. They describe PR intervals versus heart size in a spectrum of mammals ranging from the rat to the humpback whale. As the size of a mammal increases, so too does the PR interval, increasing from about 25 milliseconds in the rat to about 360 milliseconds in the horse. However, in spite of the tremendously increased size of the elephant and the humpback whale, their PR intervals remain relatively the same as that of the horse. Meijler's team notes that based on classical conduction concepts, and considering the similarity and morphological appearance of the AV node systems, it is difficult to explain why in mammals, such as whales, who have very large hearts and very large AV nodes and His-Purkinje systems, the AV transmission is not proportionately longer than in the horse. The heart weight of the humpback whale equals that of approximately two adult men and is six times the weight of an elephant heart and shows little difference in AV conduction time. In the recordings reported by Meijler's group, the heart rate of the whale is approximately 40, with a PR interval of approximately 400 milliseconds.

In a 1988 editorial published in the *Journal of the American College of Cardiology* titled, "Optimum Heart Rate of Large, Failing Hearts," Levine notes that little consideration has been given in medicine to adjusting heart rate to heart size. What, he asks, is the intrinsic heart rate of an 800-gram heart in a patient with systemic hypertension and hypertrophic or idiopathic dilated cardiomyopathy? Should the optimal heart rate for a pacemaker-dependent patient be normalized for heart size? Should we not expect a slower heart rate in patients with aortic stenosis or systemic hypertension than in patients with mild mitral valve disease?

Levine is extremely cautious about drawing conclusions from the data that he presents in his editorial, pointing out the many major constraints to the likelihood of finding a life-prolonging effect of cardiac slowing in humans. And yet, he believes that efforts to study this matter should not be discouraged. He persists in the provocative view that heart rate and life expectancy in mammals are inversely related with the product being nearly constant. This relationship, he says, prompts the question, Can human life be extended by cardiac slowing? Levine closes with the thought that an actuarial analysis of life insurance data may be of some value in trying to answer this question since a purely bradycardic agent for use in animal studies and in clinical trials is not yet available.

44

Apoptosis — the Good and the Bad: Possible Future Therapeutic Implications

September 1998

Apoptosis, a word unfamiliar to most of us just a few years ago, is now one of the hottest topics in biology. This is the observation made in a special section on apoptosis in the August 28, 1998 issue of the *Journal of Science*. An editorial in this section entitled, "Cell Death in Us and Others," by Peter Goldstein of Marseilles, France, says that while there have been scattered reports for the past century of cell death due to apoptosis, during the past five years, there have been more than 20,000 publications on apoptosis, indicating a change from mild interest to contemporary fascination.

Apoptosis is sometimes described as programmed cell death and more dramatically, as cell suicide. Apoptosis is genetically mediated cell death. In a normal animal, it is important in regulating cellularity in embryonic and adult tissues, in sculpting structures and in optimizing function in the immune and central nervous systems. Defects in these processes can result in major developmental abnormalities. In adults, apoptosis may be triggered endogenously or exogenously to turn on cell death mechanisms by evolutionarily determined death genes. Cancer or autoimmune diseases may develop when there is too little apoptosis and when there is too much, it may cause Alzheimer's disease. When ischemic stroke occurs, severely damaged cells may understandably die immediately from oxygen deprivation, but the more gradual loss of neurons in the areas outside the stroke core, when oxygen supply is reduced but not eliminated, has been a longstanding puzzle in neurology. Recent experiments in animals have found that dying cells in the periphery of the stroke area show key criteria for apoptosis. Cell death may be controlled by cystine proteases, called caspaces, that orchestrate the apoptotic process.

Writing in *Science*, Michael Moscowitz of Harvard said that it might be better to talk about caspace-mediated death. The clinical application is that caspace inhibitors, if they could be developed, may have the potential of being new pharmacological agents in the treatment of stroke. This, of course, remains to be shown. Other studies suggest that caspaces may initiate programmed cell death in Alzheimer's disease where there may be similar potential for therapeutic intervention if blocking agents for caspaces can be developed. A fascinating paper in this same issue titled, "Caspaces: Enemies Within," called apoptosis an evolutionary form of cell suicide and it delves into the role of the special machinery of the caspaces. The authors of this paper believe that ultimately, this research may result in manipulation, as they put it, of the apoptotic machinery for therapeutic gain. They echo the idea that research into the mechanisms of apoptosis will have therapeutic potential.

The medical literature is rich in studying the possible role of apoptosis in cardiovascular disease. A *New England Journal of Medicine* article in the October 1996 issue titled, "Apoptosis and Myocytes in End-Stage Heart Failure," states that while heart failure can occur from a variety of causes — including ischemia, hypertension and toxic and inflammatory diseases — the cellular mechanisms for a progressive deterioration remain unclear and may result from apoptosis. Seven patients with severe chronic heart failure were studied for evidence of apoptosis. Four had idiopathic dilated cardiomyopathy and three had ischemic cardiomyopathy. The results showed evidence of DNA laddering characteristic of apoptosis in all four patients with dilated cardiomyopathy, but not in those with ischemic cardiomyopathy. It should be remembered, of course, that reliance on a single test may be treacherous in the diagnosis of apoptosis, but based on a very few patients, the preliminary conclusion was that in end-stage dilated cardiomyopathy, apoptosis may contribute to the progressive deterioration of the ventricle.

A review article titled, "Apoptosis in Heart Failure," in the May/June 1998 issue of *Progress in Cardiovascular Disease,* comes to a similar conclusion that loss of cardiac monocytes through apoptosis may contribute to progression in heart failure. A paper in the December 1996 issue of the British *Journal of Pathology* shows that foam cell death at the edge of the lipid core in an atherosclerotic lesion is caused both by necrosis and apoptosis. The article also points out that oxidized low-density lipoproteins can cause macrophage apoptosis in vitro and may play a role in the formation and enlargement of the lipid core.

Programmed cell death or apoptosis in atherosclerosis is also described in a 1997 article in the British journal, *Heart Vessel,* which suggests the possible role of apoptosis in heart attacks and in stroke. In March 1998, the *Journal of Free Radical Biology and Medicine* published an article entitled, "Oxidative Stress Developed During Reperfusion of Ischemic Myocardium Induces Apoptosis." To determine whether is-chemic reperfusion injury is mediated by apoptotic cell death, isolated rat hearts were subjected to ischemia followed by reperfusion. The hearts processed after each experiment showed DNA laddering that was characteristic of apoptosis, suggesting that oxidative stress devel-oped in ischemic myocardial reperfusion does indeed induce apoptosis. The validity of this result is enhanced by the finding that pre-reperfu-sion pharmacological intervention prevented the appearance of post-reperfusion apoptosis. In the June 16, 1998 issue of *Circulation*, there is an article titled, "Apoptosis and Related Proteins in Different Stages of Human Atherosclerotic Plaque," by Mark Cox and his associates from Antwerp. The paper concludes that smooth muscle cells within fatty streaks express a pro-apoptotic protein that increases the susceptibility of these cells to apoptosis. The authors believe that this may be impor-tant in the transition of fatty streaks to atherosclerotic plaques. While the concept extends the ramifications of apoptosis in various disease states that may be unfamiliar territory to most of us, it is becoming ap-parent that apoptosis may play a very important role in many disease states with which we frequently deal, such as congestive heart failure, atherosclerosis, ischemic reperfusion injury and stroke.

In his editorial, Pierre Goldstein points out that cell death and the process of apoptosis cuts across a wide range of organisms and that this process has invaded not only the minds of cell biologists, but of biolo-gists in many fields. I trust that he would include physicians in his des-ignation "biologists." Goldstein states that our current understanding of the elaborate course of events within a dying cell is dominated by two major observations. The first observation, from a molecular point of view, is that cell death is the outcome of a programmed intracellular cascade of genetically determined steps, as initially shown in the nem-atode c-elegans. The second observation, from a morphological point of view, is that in animals, this cascade leads to apoptosis. Goldstein makes the strong point that apart from the sheer joy of discovery, in-vestigation of cell death or apoptosis in a spectrum of organisms may have socially beneficial applications — by which I believe he means new medical therapies.

Thus, if the process of apoptosis or programmed cell death can be understood and controlled, there may be therapeutic implications for conditions that are as diverse as cancer, Alzheimer's disease, atheroscle-rotic and ischemic syndromes and cardiomyopathies. For the control of apoptosis and its clinical application, the future may not be now, but it may well be sooner than we think.

45

On the Future of Cardiovascular Medicine and Research in the Molecular Era

August 1998

In the July 1998 issue of *Cardiovascular Research*, the journal of the European Society of Cardiology, an editorial by editor-in-chief Michiel Janse is as compelling and provocative as its title, "Quo Vadis Classical Physiology?" In October 1996, Janse had attended a lecture given by Wolfgang Schaper of the Interuniversity Cardiology Institute of the Netherlands. The lecture had begun with a slide that read, "Quo vadis classical physiology?" The next slide answered the question with the words, "Down the drain — unless it concentrates on pathophysiological mechanisms in animal models of human disease and on integrative physiology of transgenic animals."

These two slides and that lecture stimulated Dr. Janse to ask Professor Schaper to act as guest editor for the previously mentioned July 1998 issue of *Cardiovascular Research*, the thrust of which is epitomized by the title of the lead article by Schaper and Winkler: "Of Mice and Men: The Future of Cardiovascular Research in the Molecular Era." The paper begins with the observation that the molecular age "has changed experimental cardiovascular research and continues to make these changes deeper and more and more irreversible every day." According to the authors, during the last 12 years, the classic experimental animals used in cardiovascular research — dogs and cats — have become unfashionable to use for many reasons, not all of which are scientific. Some of these reasons include new legislation, great expense and interference by animal rights activists. These animals have been gradually replaced by smaller animals such as rats and rabbits, and more recently, by transgenic mice. The authors point out that this changing selection of experimental animals doesn't necessarily have its roots in new opportunities of molecular approaches. Not all cardiovascular problems can be reduced to exercises in gene expression, nor are all pharmacological problems solved using the gene approach, although screening for new pharmacological agents more and more involves genetically altered cells and animals. Gene expression research is appropriate when studying chronic adaptation of tissues to change in the environment of cells or organs, such as pressure overload or growth of new blood vessels or chronic hypoxia.

The authors emphasize that molecular biology is assuming a prominent place because it promises a paradigm shift in modern medicine, namely, that chronic degenerative diseases may be amenable to causal treatment and that structural changes may be elicited by substituting failing, weakly expressed or mutated genes. For example, the manifestations of atherosclerosis may possibly be avoided by gene therapy and existing or threatening arterial occlusions may be modified by angiogenesis and arteriogenesis. These new methods may be less expensive than surgery and traditional pharmacotherapy, and probably more socially acceptable.

The significance and relevance of the ideas expressed by Schaper and Winkler are similar to those observed by British cardiologist John Perrins, when he was interviewed at the Glasgow meeting of the British Cardiac Society by Dr. Richard Lewis of the Ohio State University School of Medicine. In that interview, Perrins said that the extent of cardiovascular disease is so great that there is political reluctance in Britain to admit its magnitude because doing so would require a great deal of money and restructuring of the way cardiac services are rendered. Perrins also said that it is a wish more than a belief that the answer to cardiovascular disease lies in primary care and prevention. Like many who deal with cardiovascular disease, Perrins doesn't really think this is true, but he believes that inevitably, we will have to deal more with older patients because our present treatment approaches slow the course of disease instead of preventing it. Therefore, today's practices will not reduce costs, but will ultimately increase the demand for resources to treat cardiovascular disease.

This concept fits very well with what Schaper and Winkler have to say. They believe that support for traditional cardiovascular research is no longer on the A list of politicians and granting agencies in Europe or in the United States, perhaps because of the enormous success enjoyed by technically oriented cardiology and cardiovascular surgery over the past 20 years. Like Perrins, Schaper and Winkler suggest that this success has created the illusion that cardiovascular disease is under control and no longer needs the generous funding that it has had for the past three decades.

Schaper and Winkler point out that another consequence of our great success in technical and instrumental solutions in cardiology is that it may have delayed the molecular approach in cardiology. In cancer research, for example, the molecular approach gained support much earlier. The authors believe that we are now on the threshold of an exciting new paradigm of biopharmacology that may very well produce structural changes in tissues by manipulation of the genome rather than by traditional acute treatment with classical pharmacology. They also suggest that the right mammalian model for future cardiovascular studies must be one that will allow manipulation of the genome. Because of expense, gestation time and technical feasibility, they believe that this is almost certainly going to be the mouse — in spite of difficulties in performing experiments in miniature. Although they may not yet be accepted as proper experimental models for the study of heart failure, hypertrophy and ischemic preconditioning, Schaper and Winkler believe that ultimately, the problems of using mice can be solved.

Much of Schaper and Winkler's paper deals with technical aspects of molecular biology, unfamiliar to many if not most clinical cardiologists (myself certainly included). But they clearly show that even to the uninitiated, cardiovascular science is at a crossroads. To them, this is invigorating — a far cry from what they call the doldrums of the mid-1980s when, in their view, new ideas were scarce and integrative cardiovascular science was being replaced by molecular sciences. They believe that a new relationship between molecular and integrative scientists will occur because both realize they cannot exist without each other. The mouse that roars, they conclude, is the heraldic animal of this new union.

If this is to occur — and it seems very likely that it will — effective communication between those in integrated cardiovascular science and those in molecular science will be paramount. This is illustrated in an article in the October 24, 1997 issue of *Science* entitled, "Functional Genomics: It's All How You Read It." The article observes that "functional genomics" is a term that is widely used (as it is in the paper by Schaper and Winkler), but that there is uncertainty as to what it really means. The article cites an informal poll among those in the field clearly showing that the term has many different interpretations. Because it is essential that the language used in scientific discourse be intelligible to all involved, responsibility is placed on readers to be informed, but also on writers to communicate with clarity.

This point is made in almost lyric prose in an article titled, "Voices of Science," by David Locke, which I came upon by chance a short time ago in *The American Scholar*. While Locke's paper deals primarily with communication by scientists to the educated public, I believe that much of what he says would also apply to dialogue between molecular and cardiovascular scientists. "The scientists, at least some of them," Locke says, "can write well, wittily, movingly and powerfully when they want to." Why then, he asks, do we see so much scientific writing that is unreadable by anyone except the six other people in the world who are working on the same set of problems? He adds that "matters will not improve until scientists are able to admit that their voices are dull, claustrophobic, confusing and alienating." As examples of scientists of more than modest achievement who did write with clarity, Locke cites the likes of Newton, Harvey, Einstein, and more recently, Watson and Crick. He suggests that the best way to improve scientific communication with the public and professionals is for writers to read the works of scientists who, even though they had something novel to say, were actually understandable. Locke's paper is stimulating, perhaps even amusing, and in it are lessons to be learned, even for those of us who may not really think of ourselves as scientists.

46

Culture and American Medicine: Puritanism, Enlightenment and the American Frontier

November 1995

Today, there are few aspects of medical practice that escape close scrutiny, but there has been little effort to explore the cultural, historical and philosophic bases for what we do and why we do it. These elements somehow seem remote to us, like vestiges of a past that we've either forgotten or failed to relate to the medicine of today. Recently, I happened upon two commentaries that bear on these very issues.

The first commentary, from *Perspectives in Biology and Medicine*, titled, "Culture and Medicine: The Influence of Puritanism on American Medical Practice," is written by James Goodwin from the Center on Aging at the University of Texas at Galveston. Dr. Goodwin observes that during a period of rapid transition in medicine, it should not be forgotten that everything we do occurs in a cultural context. He points out that scientific medicine is virtually the same in the United States as it is in Western Europe and that American, Italian, German, Swedish or French scientists working on DNA, for example, would be as comfortable in a laboratory in New York City as in Rome or Paris. And because there is a universal language for scientific medicine — English — communication is very easy.

There are, however, huge differences in the way medicine is practiced in the United States and other countries, differences that Goodwin feels can be attributed to our culture and heritage. He illustrates this with a comparison of the ten most widely prescribed medications in the United States and in several Western European countries during the late 1970s. In the United States, three of the top ten agents prescribed were sedatives and hypnotics and the rest were antibiotics, anti-inflammatories and anti-hypertensives. In France, liver preparations topped the list and in Italy, five of the most frequently prescribed medicines were hormones. He also notes that German doctors prescribed many of their medications by rectal suppository instead of orally. Today, in the United States, a patient with malaise is likely to be considered nervous, depressed or perhaps the victim of a virus, but in France, this same malaise is frequently attributed to a liver problem. In Germany and in other continental countries, low blood pressure is an accepted diagnosis that is frequently used to explain fatigue, while in the United States and in Britain, it is considered a "disreputable diagnosis," to use Goodwin's words.

Goodwin advances the thesis that Puritanism is such a deeply ingrained part of American culture that even today, it influences our attitude toward medicine. The tenets of Puritanism that Goodwin describes include that life is serious, earnest and grim and that external manifestations of pleasure are always somewhat suspect. He cites four examples where remnants of this philosophy may still influence the American approach to medicine.

The first concerns alcohol and our tendency to minimize what he calls compelling epidemiological evidence that moderate alcohol consumption may reduce the incidence of coronary artery disease. Goodwin believes that our reluctance to accept the potential benefits of alcohol, even in moderate amounts, despite the epidemiological data, may be cultural rather than scientific. The next example concerns the alleviation of pain and the reluctance of American physicians to prescribe pain medication. This issue is the subject of the recent Agency for Healthcare Policy and Research Guidelines for physicians and nurses that were created to overcome what the AHCPR perceives to be the under-utilization of narcotics and analgesics in hospitalized patients, postoperative patients and even those with terminal cancer. Goodwin believes that "no program to promote the humane treatment of people in pain can hope to succeed if it addresses only the scientific issues such as pharmacokinetics and ignores the value that our culture places on asceticism."

The third area is pregnancy. Goodwin believes that the puritanical attitude toward pregnancy, which can be described as uncomfortable at best, may be responsible in part for the way in which, over the past 100 years, American medicine has redefined pregnancy and childbirth from a natural process to a pathological one. He also believes that Puritanism may influence medicine's abstemious approach to the management of pregnancy, which until recently, rigorously controlled weight gain. Goodwin also feels that the absolute interdiction of even minimal amounts of alcohol during all phases of pregnancy may be more cultural than scientific.

Finally, Goodwin feels that it is not difficult to recognize the strong Puritanism in the American preventive medicine movement, noting that the fervor for reducing cholesterol in the United States is unmatched in most European countries. While Goodwin finds no fault with preventive measures such as dietary restriction, prohibition of smoking and advocacy of weight loss and exercise, he believes that there is a puritanical selectivity in emphasis. For example, he cites substantive evidence that marriage and the avoidance of social isolation will increase longevity and protect against various diseases, yet he sees little promotion of marriage as a preventive health measure. Goodwin feels that in general, European cultures do not see asceticism as the worthy public health goal that he believes it is in the United States.

The second commentary, an interesting companion piece to the Goodwin article, is a paper published in March 1995 in the *Mayo Clinic Proceedings* entitled, "Influences of American Philosophy and History on the Practice of American Medicine," written by Dr. Stephen Weiss of Eau Clair, Wisconsin. Like Goodwin, Weiss believes that cultural factors, such as historical experiences and philosophic traditions, affect the way American physicians practice medicine. Paramount among these are the three basic concepts of American Enlightenment philosophy — reason, experience and progress. Weiss quotes Benjamin Franklin, whom he calls one of the apostles of the American Enlightenment, who said, "I have long been so impressed by the invention and acquisition of new and useful utensils and instruments, that I have sometimes almost wished that it had been my destiny to be born two or three centuries hence — for invention and improvement are prolific and beget more of their kind." No doubt, Franklin was correct in wishing that he had been born 200 years later. How he would have relished our current science and technology, especially in medicine.

The British historian and statesman, James Bryce, praised the exuberance of America's West, saying that it was already living in the future, with today only half finished and yesterday already forgotten. Weiss contends that American frontier philosophy — ever moving forward with no thought of failure, with no goal being insurmountable — is part of the philosophy of American medical technology that advances even more rapidly than our understanding of how best to use it. Thus, our historic and philosophic bias in favor of new technology epitomizes the practice of American medicine. These influences are profound and seem to clash with the restrictions and restraints imposed by managed care. Weiss describes our American history as one of a people on the move — a people who believe that any goal can be achieved. There is little patience for the status quo. Medicine is suffused with what I would call a can-do frontier philosophy that underlies its lust for action and innovation. Thus, three somewhat contradictory elements in our past — Puritan asceticism, boundless Enlightenment optimism and frontier energy — have defined American medicine and influence it still.

47

Remembering Irvine Page

August 1991

On June 10th of this year, death claimed one of America's great physician-scientists, Dr. Irvine Page. Dr. Page was 90 when he died of a heart attack, an event that he had experienced for the first time in 1967. I had the privilege of knowing Dr. Page and spending some time with him on several different occasions. Like many great men, he had that faculty for putting ordinary people at ease. He was a raconteur whose conversations sparkled with wit and humor. He was incisive and not hesitant to take a stand.

Irvine Page studied biochemistry at Cornell where he later received his medical degree. He was a house officer at Belleview and at Presbyterian Hospital in New York City and he directed the Chemical Division of the Kaiser Wilhelm Institute in Munich where he became interested in neurochemistry. After a time at the Rockefeller Institute in New York, he went on to Indianapolis where he was in change of the Lilly Laboratory for Clinical Research. In 1945, he began a 21-year tour at the Cleveland Clinic Foundation, ultimately making it a leading research center, particularly in the areas of high blood pressure and heart disease. Dr. Page also conducted seminal work in the discovery of angiotensin and serotonin, which he and his associates later synthesized.

In 1961, Dr. Page became the editor of *Modern Medicine*, to which he contributed dozens of editorials, many of which were collected in 1972 in a delightful volume. When he became editor, he stated that his purpose was "to cover as broad an area as possible and to bring to [the journal] a degree of honesty, even if it hurts." Dr. Page not only said these words, he lived by them. Dr. Page believed in the individual. He didn't much like corporate medicine or medicine as a business, a trend that was just getting under way during his active years as editor. But he was perceptive and recognized what was about to happen. The titles of his essays give the flavor of his thinking. One was called, "The New Conglomerate, Washington Itself." A few of the words from his essay make his point: "The growth of power in this new Washington conglomerate is its frightening aspect. I know many persons there and almost none of them are aware of how the capital scene has changed them. The atmosphere of adulation being taken seriously, special small privileges, not being contradicted in making decisions that shake the country's foundation, is a heady environment. Few can withstand it and almost everyone wants to be exposed to it."

Dr. Page was outraged by the growing role of the media in medicine. I wonder what he would say today. He wrote an article called, "The Partial Truth Syndrome," in which he objected to "creating celebrities almost by Madison Avenue methods in both science and medicine," and in the same essay, he observed, "Skepticism and truth are inseparable companions. When people become fearful and silence the skeptic, the world of the intellect is in trouble." On ethics, Dr. Page drove his point home when he said, "Our ethics must include ways of dealing with the mass media without allowing medicine to be dragged into the commotion of the market place." Little did he know how prophetic his words would be; there is no doubt that we are now indeed practicing medicine in the marketplace.

Dr. Page's thinking also comes through in an essay he called, "Obfuscation by Planning," in which he said: "Basic research, a delicate process, [is] easily snuffed out and often influenced by the environment of the laboratory. The creative mind, especially if it is not the best — and that describes most of us — can be inhibited. Complex apparatus, large technical staffs, grant requests, committee reports, travel to meetings and struggle of public recognition, all are distractions." Dr. Page illustrates this by saying that if Alexander Fleming had had a committee and a modern laboratory, he surely would never have discovered penicillin. Perhaps things were simpler then. Dr. Page did grow up in another world, but the truths that he held are universal and perhaps needed more today than in his own time.

Dr. Page once wrote an essay called, "Death with Dignity," in which he said, "All reasonable efforts should be made to stay death, but there are unreasonable efforts as well. Man should still have the right to die at home among those he loves." And this is exactly what Irvine Page did in Hyannisport, Massachusetts, just a few weeks ago. Few of us will ever match the accomplishments of Dr. Page, but in a time when there seem to be fewer and fewer heroes, surely he is one to remember and to emulate. "Role model" has become a hackneyed expression, but if you are in search of one, review the career and writings of Dr. Irvine Page.

48

The Propriety of Promotional Marketing of Technologies in Progress

April 1997

The current status of minimally invasive bypass surgery and also its future prospects was the subject of one of the plenary debates last month at the scientific sessions of the American College of Cardiology in Anaheim, California. Although several forms of so-called minimalist approaches to bypass surgery are now in the process of development, they are still works in progress and have yet to find their place in the pantheon of accepted cardiovascular surgical techniques. This uncertain current status has not, however, deterred extensive promotional marketing. To illustrate this, I will quote from an advertisement promoting minimally invasive bypass surgery that was played on the radio throughout the Nashville area:

> "If you or someone you know is a candidate for heart surgery, consider this. Most open heart surgery begins with a foot-long incision, then the patient's chest bone is cut in half, and then the heart is stopped. From that point on, it's a race against time. But at Columbia Centennial, doctors can now perform open heart surgery in some patients through an incision less than four inches long, with no broken chest bone and without stopping the heart. Open heart surgery with faster recovery, less risk and less cost. And here's something else to consider. Columbia Centennial was the first hospital in Tennessee to offer this advanced heart surgery. If you're experiencing heart problems or if you just want more information, get to the heart of the matter. Call Columbia today at 1-800 Columbia."

Simultaneously, in Nashville newspapers, large ads appeared headlining: "Doctors at Columbia Centennial were the First in the Area to Perform Open Heart Surgery Through an Incision This Big." Below these bold-faced words appeared a short, slightly curved dotted line representing the incision. Beneath this drawing, the ad continues, "Instead of a large incision through the breastbone, Columbia physicians now conduct bypass surgery through an incision less than four inches long. With minimally invasive coronary artery bypass surgery, we can operate on a beating heart, so eligible patients are no longer routinely placed on a heart/lung machine. Faster recovery, less risk and less cost."

The Nashville radio and newspaper ads touting surgical technologies that are still under development and as yet not proven, are prime examples of medical advertising for commercial and promotional purposes. Once the object of disapproval and derision by doctors, advertising is now unfortunately commonplace in our most prestigious, respected and venerable medical institutions. Yet the propriety of promoting as state-of-the-art those procedures that are still being defined and developed and even those that are experimental is a matter that should be of concern to doctors and patients alike.

"Irrational exuberance" (a phrase that usually refers to investor overconfidence) and hyperbole in medical advertising reflect negatively on the doctors who will be performing these procedures. They cannot avoid at least some responsibility for how their work is being promulgated and advertised to the public.

49

Industry, Academia and the
Medical Literature

May 1997

In the *Journal of the American Medical Association* for April 16, 1997, there is a paper titled, "Bioequivalence of Generic and Brand-name Levothyroxine Products in the Treatment of Hypothyroidism." Ordinarily, this rather uninspiring title would surely not have attracted much attention, except perhaps for a glance at the conclusion that the generic and brand-name forms of levothyroxine are, by current FDA criteria, bioequivalent and interchangeable as a thyroid replacement for most patients — and even then, it's not terribly exciting. But the article by Dr. Betty Dong and her associates from the University of California at San Francisco (UCSF) is far more important than might appear from its title and the events relating to and preceding its publication are far more important to medical journalism than just a comparison of brand-name and generic levothyroxine.

In the April 26, 1997 issue of the *New York Times*, under the title, "Experts See Bias in Drug Data," the well-known medical writer, Lawrence Altman, himself a doctor, explores the history and implications of the Dong paper. Altman opens by setting the stage for a penetrating analysis that should be of great interest to those engaged in medical research who accept grants from industry and to doctors who practice medicine and depend on the medical literature. "Suppression of a university scientist's findings about a common thyroid drug by a company that paid for the research," he comments, "has raised serious questions about how the growing link between industry and academia affects the reliability of information provided to doctors and to the public about drugs and other therapies." Altman notes that in recent years, while medical leaders have been troubled by the reluctance of scientists and journal editors to publish negative studies, little attention has been given to the way in which contracts between industry and academia may influence what gets published. The publication of Dong's seemingly innocuous paper has brought this influence under close scrutiny.

In the same issue of *JAMA*, there is an editorial titled, "Thyroid Storm," by Drummond Rennie, a deputy editor of the journal. He describes the astounding series of events that led to the delayed publication of the levothyroxine paper. Dr. Dong's research project actually began some nine years earlier, when Flint Laboratories, then the manufacturer of the levothyroxine Synthroid, sought to compare their product with competing preparations. They fully expected it to show superiority. But this was not the case. According to an article in the April 25, 1997 issue of *Science*, when Dr. Dong showed the results to Flint's successor, Boots Pharmaceutical, that company charged that the study was seriously flawed and complained to the UCSF chancellor and several department heads. Despite this, university investigators found no reason to deny publication and the article was submitted to *JAMA*. Five referees, some with ties to Boots, found the paper to be acceptable and after minor revisions, *JAMA* scheduled publication for January 1995. But less than two weeks before publication, UCSF lawyers asked Dr. Dong to withdraw her paper because the contract she had signed with Boots Pharmaceutical gave the company veto power over publication.

Dong conceded that she had been naive to sign the contract but that a now-retired UCSF lawyer had advised her that the university would be able to get around the power to veto publication clause. But now, there was a new attorney at the UCSF and he concluded that the contract was indeed binding and that the university would not defend the authors if they were sued. The Chairman of the Biopharmaceutical Science Department at UCSF, who had tried to mediate the problem between the author and Boots, said that the university (and again I'm quoting from *Science)* "fell down in its responsibility" to the faculty and to the public. In the meantime, Boots presented its own analysis of Dr. Dong's data in a new publication called the *American Journal of Therapeutics*. Entitled, "Limitations of Levothyroxine Bioequivalency Evaluation: Analysis of an Attempted Study," the paper did not mention Dong at all. On April 25, 1996, the *Wall Street Journal* was the first to break the story on how Boots used its contractual veto power to stop publication of a paper that had already been accepted by *JAMA* and how they forced UCSF to acquiesce with threats of a protracted lawsuit.

This episode has attracted a tremendous amount of attention including a July 26, 1996 editorial in *Science* aptly titled, "A Cautionary Tale," in which Dorothy Zinberg of the Kennedy School of Government at Harvard quoted former Harvard President Derrick Bok, who said in a seminar on university-industry relations that the "price of corporate support is eternal vigilance." In her editorial, Zinberg called the UCSF-Boots episode a morality play that gives substance to Bok's warning that corporations considering less than disinterested research sponsorship should ponder the long-term consequences of their actions. Zinberg added that the *Wall Street Journal's* early warning came none too soon.

The long delay in publishing Dr. Dong's article and the accompanying editorial by Dr. Drummond Rennie that detailed the story behind the efforts of the pharmaceutical sponsor to prevent publication have reverberated around the world. The *Wall Street Journal* and the *New York Times* and *Science* were not alone in reporting this event. The *British Medical Journal* for April 19, 1997 recounted the legal maneuverings that led to the seven-year delay in publication and they repeated Rennie's warning that investigators should not assume that sponsors will encourage publication of unfavorable results and that they should never be allowed veto power. Richard Horton, the editor of the *Lancet*, said that journals need to be more aware of who owns the data, perhaps referring to the article by Boots in the *American Journal of Therapeutics* that presented its own interpretation of Dong's data.

No one seems to know how often restrictive contracts are written. Dr. Mary Pendergast, a Deputy Commissioner of the Food and Drug Administration, with whom I spoke about this matter, said that the FDA sees only the data and not the contracts and has no way of knowing how often such agreements prevent publication by academic investigators. She did say, however, that the data seen by the FDA are often not consistent with the far rosier picture portrayed when the material is actually published in the scientific literature. Altman suggests that federal health officials, university faculty members, drug companies and journal editors consider this particular case to be unusual. Others, however, say that there are few ways to determine how often a work is not published because of restrictive contracts. For finally publishing the UCSF paper and for offering Dr. Rennie's candid editorial exposing the history of this attempt to suppress publication, *JAMA* deserves great credit as does the *Wall Street Journal* for first bringing this episode to public scrutiny. Subsequent coverage and analysis by the *New York Times, Science,* the *British Medical Journal,* the *Lancet,* and perhaps other publications of which I'm not aware, once again prove the vital role of a free and investigative press. Even scientific journals, to their great credit, are beginning to assume an investigative role in areas that affect medical research, practice and scientific journalism.

The title of the July 1996 editorial in *Science* — "A Cautionary Tale" — is appropriate, but perhaps understated. This tale is more than cautionary, it's frightening. We all trust and want to believe that the suppression of the Dong paper is a rare case. But for the sake of academic and scientific integrity, and to preserve trust in the medical literature, restrictive agreements giving industry influence and veto power over publication must be outlawed. And yet, in an imperfect world where ulterior motives and secret agendas may occur even in the laboratory, the academy and in the board room, the investigator, the reviewer, the editor — and perhaps even more important, the reader — might well put skepticism before trust.

50

The Media and Managed Care

April 1998

In the January/February 1998 issue of *Health Affairs*, there is a cover story entitled, "Media Coverage of Managed Care: Is There a Negative Bias?" by Mollyanne Brodie and Drew Altman, who hold doctorates in health policy and political science, and by Lee Ann Brady, Director of Media Analysis Studies at Princeton Research Associates in New Jersey. Their article analyzes print and broadcast media reporting of the managed care industry from January 1, 1990, through June 30, 1997. The authors tell us that managed care dominates the U.S. health-care market — something that we all know. I didn't know — and perhaps I'm not alone in this — that there was a rise in the adoption of managed care coverage in businesses with more than 200 employees from 29 percent in 1988 to 81 percent in 1997. More than a third of the 35 million Medicaid beneficiaries are enrolled in managed care health plans and the Congressional Budget Office projects that by the year 2007, a third of Medicare's 30 million beneficiaries will be as well.

To achieve a broad view of the media coverage of managed care, the authors reviewed *USA Today*, *The Wall Street Journal*, the *New York Times*, the *Los Angeles Times*, the *Cleveland Plain Dealer* and the *Orlando Sentinel* and two magazines, *Forbes* and *Business Week*. Using Lexis-Nexis and Dow Jones databases, they found and analyzed some 2100 articles pertinent to managed care. They also analyzed broadcast news stories from ABC, CBS and NBC, which they acquired from the Vanderbilt University Television News Archives.

In their review, the authors found that from 1990 to 1997, the media coverage of managed care gradually shifted its emphasis from business issues to policy and politics and more recently, to the growing backlash against managed care. In 1990, 9 percent of the media reports on managed care concerned political and legislative issues. By 1993, these topics increased to 34 percent of the coverage, but by 1996, they had dropped to only 11 percent. Gradually, the emphasis shifted to patients and consumer protection, so that by 1997, these subjects comprised 44 percent of the media reports.

The attitude of the press also changed. In 1990 and 1991, journalists portrayed HMOs as villains 7 to 12 percent of the time and by 1997, 20 percent of journalists were critical of managed care and only 4 percent had positive things to say. When the topic of coverage concerned the way in which managed care handled medical care, 45 percent of journalists were either neutral or critical and 9 percent were positive.

All things considered, the authors conclude that media coverage itself is not responsible for creating the managed care backlash that exists today. They point out that while their study examines the nature of media coverage, it does not address the more fundamental issue of whether the media portrayals of managed care — positive or negative — actually reflect reality. It seems to me that the implication and tone of their paper is that media coverage has become more critical over time, not because of media bias, but because of what is actually happening in the industry.

In the same issue of *Health Affairs*, there is an article entitled, "Covering a Breaking Revolution: The Media and Managed Care," by Karen Ignagni, Chief Executive of the American Association of Health Plans. Ignagni suggests that critics of managed care have become adroit at selectively publicizing managed care's alleged failure to deliver service. She feels that these events are amplified by the media and tend to become the basis for legislation in the name of consumer protection. Not surprisingly, Ignagni says that journalists know that a well-administered health plan promotes optimal care at affordable cost by ensuring that patients get the right care at the right time in the right setting.

Ignagni believes that the media is susceptible to charges that health plans contain costs by denying referrals, limiting access to high-cost treatments and being otherwise stingy with care. She claims that these charges are unwarranted because the criticism levied against "drive-through deliveries," outpatient mastectomies and gag rules for physicians is, in her opinion, unfair. On the gag rule issue, Ignagni states that such rules do not exist. "Given the historical sanctity of the doctor/patient relationship, it would be hard to imagine how health plans could contemplate, let alone perpetrate, such an obvious breach of ethics." She goes on to say that the General Accounting Office in Washington has reported that health plans are doing no such thing. She contends that gag rules exist only "in the minds of critics who have no compunction about distorting the true purpose of clauses that protect the confidentiality of financial statements or disparagement of a plan by a physician contracting with competing plans." According to Ignagni, the gag rule "myth" is finally on its way to oblivion. She laments that a national news magazine with a circulation of millions featured a muzzled doctor on its cover. She bemoans the 32 states that have passed laws protecting "consumers" against this "non-threat." Ignagni denies the existence of drive-through deliveries and regarding the criticism of too-short stays for breast cancer surgery, she says it is made by critics who, in her mind, are not distinguishing between lumpectomies and mastectomies. Ignagni likens the charges the media makes against managed care to crying "fire" in a crowded theater. She defends managed care as work in progress and believes that policymakers and legislators must decide whether to encourage this work in progress or put on the brakes.

Ignagni thinks it is still not widely understood that health plans make business decisions within the context of doing what is best for patients. She claims that "putting patients first" is not only a motto for managed care, but a mission that is explicit in the code of professional ethics that has been adopted by more than 1000 American associations of health plan members, who, to maintain membership in the plan, must continue to adhere to this ethical statement. Ignagni believes that those in the legislative arena have limited ability to evaluate allocations of substandard care and she inveighs against congressional and state legislators who produce measures that can lead to what she calls governmental micromanagement. From Ignagni's article, it is obvious that she considers any attempt by Congress or state legislators to regulate or restrain managed care as governmental micromanagement. Micromanagement of medical care should therefore, I presume, remain the unchallenged province of the managed care industry.

It is with reluctance that I have to express some disappointment with John Iglehart's introductory editorial to the two papers that I have just reviewed. Under the title, "The Media as Messenger," Iglehart describes the media's reporting of managed care as mixed and confused. About the Brodie, Altman and Brady paper analyzing media coverage of managed care, he says, "what our lead paper does not cover is [that] important stories that would cast managed care in a more favorable light tend to be neglected." He claims that managed care has received little credit for what he calls "systemic improvements" in the quality of care. On the other hand, he praises Ignagni and her paper for what he calls her "splendid suggestion" that health plan organizations invite journalists inside to witness how they identify the best practices and partner with providers and patients to promote continuous quality improvement. About Ignagni's offer to show reporters the inside workings of managed care, Inglehart says, "Her prescription is a therapeutic formula for reporters, particularly those who regard health plans as less than forthright about how they allocate resources within their fixed budgets."

It is unfortunate that John Iglehart, the very highly regarded editor of *Health Affairs*, selected Ignagni to critique the media analysis paper, considering that as the spokesperson for the managed care industry, she is hardly an unbiased observer. Iglehart's choice might have been acceptable had he also printed an analysis by someone with a less-vested interest in managed care than Ignagni. In addition, Inglehart's own bias comes through quite clearly in his editorial when he criticizes the media for pushing provocative issues and for not providing appropriate balance in its managed care coverage.

I believe that the most statesmanlike message in these three articles comes from the authors of "Media Coverage and Managed Care," when they say that the performance of managed care has had such an important impact on Americans that managed care is receiving and warrants great attention. They continue, "the media coverage merits monitoring in the future, but for now, it seems wise to focus on the real pros and cons of managed care rather than on media performance." Today it is popular in Washington for institutions, organizations and individuals to defend against criticism of their performance by blaming media coverage. In defending managed care so absolutely, both Iglehart and Ignagni are clearly adhering to this tradition.

51

Scientific Journalism in the Marketplace

June 1998

In the *New York Times Magazine* of June 28, 1998 there is an article that casts a somewhat jaundiced eye on some of the practices of our best known and widely read medical publications — the *New England Journal of Medicine* and the *Journal of the American Medical Association*. The article is entitled, "The Hippocratic Wars: The Feisty *Journal of the American Medical Association* and the Staid *New England Journal of Medicine* are Battling for Physician-Readers Through an Unwitting Ally — The Media," written by Ellen Ruppel Shell, co-director of the science journalism program at Boston University.

Shell takes *JAMA* to task for the way it promoted a January 7, 1998 paper called, "Fish Consumption and Risk of Sudden Death" based on the U.S. Physicians Health Study. Prior to *JAMA's* publication of this paper, according to Shell, "the AMA press office deluged 2500 media outlets around the world with press packets, emails, faxes, and for broadcasters [they provided] tantalizing chunks of ready-to-air film footage trumpeting the findings of the study —a link between fish consumption and a 52 percent reduction in sudden cardiac death." As she anticipated, "this [media] effort had the desired effect." The fish and sudden death story was covered extensively by ABC, CNN, *Time* magazine, the *Washington Post*, the *New York Times*, and by the foreign press from Ireland to Asia. Major wire services and radio networks also ran the story. A restaurant trade journal reported a spike in fish sales and that fishmongers planned a new advertising slogan: "Seafood. Take It to Heart."

The *JAMA* fish consumption article seems far less impressive than the press releases and the subsequent coverage by the media. Using data from the well-known Physicians Health Study, it reported on some 20,000 male physicians, 90 percent of whom reported eating fish one or more times a week. This information was obtained from the subjects at intervals over an 11-year period. There were 133 sudden deaths during the course of the study. After controlling for age, randomized aspirin and beta-carotene consumption and coronary risk factors, the study found that among those who ate fish at least once a week, the relative risk of sudden death was 0.48 with a 95 percent confidence interval, compared with men who consumed fish less than once a month. The fish intake was not associated with the reduced risk of total MI, non-sudden cardiac death or total cardiovascular mortality, but was associated only with a reduced all-cause mortality. The article concluded, "These prospective data suggest that consumption of fish at least once a week may reduce the risk of sudden cardiac death in men."

Accompanying the *JAMA* article on fish consumption is an editorial by Daan Kromhout, a researcher with the National Institute of Public Health in the Netherlands. Kromhout notes that in the five years since he initially reported that the once- or twice-weekly consumption of fish caused a 50 percent reduction in coronary heart disease mortality, the controversy surrounding this association has been increased by the publication of negative results in two large cohort studies in the United States and by inconsistent findings in three other studies. Kromhout's editorial also emphasizes that in the Physicians Health Study, the men who ate fish less frequently also had more risk factors for sudden death than the men with a higher fish intake. They smoked more, drank more alcohol and exercised less. He notes that although the authors had adjusted for these risk factors, residual confounding elements remained. And Shell's article suggests that the *JAMA* report may have been nothing more than a statistical fluke. Although Shell criticized the *JAMA* press releases for not emphasizing the caveats in Kromhout's editorial, she did not mention that he also suggested that there was evidence that fish consumption once a week might help prevent coronary disease and, therefore, it should be a component of a healthy diet. Thus even though it criticizes the press releases, the Shell article did not cover Kromhout's editorial adequately.

George Lundberg, editor of *JAMA*, didn't seem to consider promotion of the fish consumption article a problem, and when confronted with the highly questionable quality of the paper, he answered rather cavalierly, "People are told that eating fish once a week is not a bad thing," and with a shrug added, "What harm could it do?" Presumably, presenting to the public as definitive information that is still open to considerable controversy and making it into a media event is not important to Lundberg.

Shell then turned her attention to Dr. Jerome Kassirer, editor-in-chief of the *New England Journal of Medicine*. She had asked him what his journal had in the pipeline. Kassirer quite properly declined to discuss upcoming articles, but did hint that he and Marcia Angell, his executive editor, had a special editorial planned for the New Year's edition. This editorial, to be titled, "Losing Weight: An Ill-fated New Year's Resolution," would encourage Americans not to sacrifice one of the great pleasures of life — eating. When it appeared, the editorial apparently led to a spate of letters to the editor charging that the journal had trivialized obesity, the second leading cause of preventable death in the United States. When Shell asked Angell if she found this criticism unsettling, Angell smiled and said, "Given the choice, we prefer not to be boring."

To this comment, Shell responded that, in truth, neither the *New England Journal* nor *JAMA* could afford to be boring and that the competition for subscribers, advertising dollars and intellectual primacy between these two eminent medical journals is fierce. While both journals have a distinguished history of publishing landmark research, she added, such papers have very little "marquee value" and for this reason, they also tend to publish "tantalizing and suggestive research on sex, food, exercise and lifestyle breakthroughs." If editors have their eye on media coverage, it's perhaps inevitable — even if at a subliminal level — that they will lean toward publishing articles likely to have appeal to the broadcast and print media. Shell gives as an example a *New England Journal* article appearing in the January 8, 1998 issue, stating that walking two miles a day cut in half the death rate of a group of men between 61 and 81 years old. As suggested by several letters to the editor on this subject, this paper may have also presented an overly sanguine view of how walking two miles a day can reduce mortality. Shell's article shows how strongly that paper was played by the press. In all fairness, the media attention may not have been because the *New England Journal* promoted the paper to the press, although perhaps the journal did not distinguish itself by publishing the article in the first place.

Lawrence Altman, MD, a veteran medical reporter with the *New York Times*, is quoted by Shell as follows: "Lundberg, the *JAMA* editor, courts the press for the same reasons that everyone else does — because he wants publicity to attract advertising." Just how far Lundberg will go is demonstrated by his publication in the April 1, 1998 *JAMA* of an article called, "Debunking Therapeutic Touch," that deals with an alternative medicine technique taught in many nursing schools. One of the authors was Linda Rosa, a nurse and member of the National Council Against Health Fraud. The other author was her 11-year-old daughter, Emily, who reportedly designed her test of therapeutic touch as a fourth-grade science project. The article received tremendous coverage in *Time* magazine and on CBS, CNN and NBC. Emily was billed as the youngest person ever to publish in the prestigious *Journal of the*

American Medical Association. Lundberg admitted the article wouldn't have made it through peer review five years ago, but he made no apologies for running it or for his lavish courtship of the press.

JAMA routinely sends out thousands of promotional copies to journalists along with press packets that highlight the week's "hot stories." In addition, a 2 1/2-minute video accessible by satellite is made available to every TV network and station in the country. Neal Freeman, Chairman of the Blackwell Corporation, which produces the weekly Public Broadcasting System television series *Technopolitics*, says that these *JAMA* releases are designed to deceive viewers by making press puffery look like journalism. Jerome Kassirer contends that he has no interest in making news and cites as evidence the fact that his journal, the *New England Journal of Medicine*, has turned down noteworthy papers that later appeared in *JAMA* to great fanfare. Kassirer states categorically that the *New England Journal* does not and never will circulate news releases and doesn't even have a news office — a position for which I believe Kassirer and his journal deserve great credit. Shell said that the very mention of video news releases made Kassirer's upper lip curl. Eight years ago, when the *New England Journal*, which was published on Thursday, appeared to be getting more than its share of news coverage, *JAMA* moved its publication date from Friday to Wednesday. This move was most likely calculated to help *JAMA* get to the public media before the *New England Journal*.

Reporters and the media are not merely conduits for information from medical journals. In a sense, the mainstream press has become something of a watchdog of the scientific medical press. Two years ago, when the *New England Journal* published an editorial claiming that the benefits of the anti-obesity drug, dexfenfluramine, outweighed its risks and that it was an important advance in the clinician's arsenal, the *Wall Street Journal* and the *New York Times* reported that the authors of that editorial served as consultants for the drug's manufacturer and distributor. The *New England Journal* editors called this an unfortunate but atypical occurrence.

Ellen Ruppel Shell's *New York Times* article is important because it raises a legitimate question about how far scientific medical journals should go in publicizing their material to the public. The policy of the *New England Journal* not to issue press releases may well be the high road. It should be the responsibility of the press to cull what is noteworthy and newsworthy from scientific publications. Also, the press always has access to consultants in medicine, just as it does in every other field from the military, to space exploration, and to areas of science and technology just as sophisticated as medicine. Referring to the original articles and using medical consultants is much more likely to result in a candid and critical analysis of medical journal papers than is achieved by relying only on press releases issued by the publisher. But even this approach has its limitations. For example, when I went back to the medical journals that Shell cited in her *New York Times* article, I realized that her presentation of those articles was somewhat misleading and slanted. But even allowing for this shortcoming, going back to the source is better than relying only on publisher press releases.

During the past two decades, the marketplace has changed medicine irrevocably, both in the practice and in the academy. Perhaps these market forces were inexorable and beyond the control of the profession. But this is probably not true in the case of medical scientific journalism, which seems to have entered the marketplace willingly, perhaps cynically and for all the wrong reasons. The interest in potential media coverage may explain why medical journal editors are so willing, if not eager, to print papers that claim such an extravagant reduction in sudden death from eating fish and in mortality in older men who walk two miles a day.

52

Reflections on Advocacy:
Ethics and Limits

May 2000

oday's practice of medicine is unique in that doctors must not only make therapeutic and diagnostic decisions, but because of the limitations and constraints imposed by the managed care-insurance complex, they are faced with an increasingly challenging and ambiguous role in implementing these decisions. The measures to which doctors have resorted to get what they consider appropriate care for their patients are the subject of a timely and significant article entitled, "Physician Manipulation of Reimbursement Rules for Patients," in the April 12, 2000 issue of the *Journal of the American Medical Association*. The lead author of the paper is Matthew K. Wynia from the AMA Institute for Ethics and the New England Medical Center Division of Clinical Care Research.

This study derives from the observation that health plans, driven by an imperative to lower costs and to maximize profits, alter and limit the medical services that doctors give to their patients. It has been suspected that some physicians, as a result of these measures, have chosen to manipulate the rules, but the extent to which this is done is not known. To find this out is, in essence, the purpose of Wynia's 1998 study.

A random sample of some 1124 doctors was obtained from the AMA master file of doctors practicing in the United States. Sixty-four percent of the doctors responded, yielding a study cohort of 720 practicing doctors. An independent survey research firm, the National Opinion Research Center at the University of Chicago, conducted all of the mailings and phone calls, thus assuring that neither the individuals nor their health plans could be identified. The study identified three devices by which doctors tried to get the coverage they deemed necessary for optimal care of their patients. These devices were exaggerating the severity of a patient's condition, modifying a patient's diagnosis and reporting signs and symptoms that the patient did not have.

All practicing physicians are well aware that utilization review, before, during and after the fact, may involve diagnostic tests, interventions and hospitalizations. This is viewed by many doctors as excessive, time-consuming and an undue challenge to their autonomy. Doctors are torn between their professional obligation as advocates for their patients and conflicting, vague and at times unacceptable contractual restraints imposed by third parties. The authors suggest that some insurers are "gaming" the system for both patients and doctors by routinely denying coverage and then approving services on subsequent appeal, knowing that time and other constraints will prevent many, if not most, of those appeals. To retaliate, doctors can be tempted to turn the tables by manipulating utilization rules so that they can get necessary medical services for their patients. To some, this may seem like manipulation, but to many doctors it is patient advocacy and indeed their professional duty.

The survey showed that 39 percent of the 720 doctors surveyed said that sometimes, often, or very often they exaggerate the severity of the patient's condition, change the diagnosis, or report symptoms that the patient didn't have. More than half of the doctors reported that they use these tactics more often now than they did five years ago. And more than one-fourth agreed that it was necessary to game the system to provide patients with high-quality care.

To find out whether doctors consider gaming the system a legitimate part of patient advocacy, Wynia's team asked three questions. First, is it ethical to game the system for your patient's benefit? Second, is it a physician's responsibility to advocate for the patient, even if it involves, for example, exaggerating severity of the patient's condition? And third, assuming that the intent is good and in the patient's interest, is exaggerating the facts an acceptable practice?

The 39 percent of doctors who used at least one such tactic during the past year were compared with those who rarely or never did. Those who gamed the system — a ratio of 3.7 compared to those who did not — believed that it was necessary to provide high-quality care. But even among this group, while some believed that it was ethically acceptable, the majority did not. This may reflect the position of the AMA and other medical organizations that have consistently opposed the manipulation of utilization, regardless of intent. Wynia and his co-authors believe that neither ethical pronouncements nor further fraud and abuse enforcement is likely to deter manipulation of utilization by doctors who see this as the only way to provide high-quality care to their patients. Furthermore, the authors found evidence suggesting that financial self-interest was not the major motivation for most doctors who manipulated reimbursement and utilization rules. They found, for example, that there was no association between this kind of activity and financial markers such as proportion of income at risk, type of reimbursement (whether fee-for-service or capitation), salary and recent practice income loss.

Doctors are caught in a kind of catch-22 between adhering to third-party limits on their options for treating patients and at the same time being liable for failure to deliver high-quality medical care. While the authors admit that neither their study nor any study can answer the question, "When, if ever, is it good for a contract to be broken in a surreptitious act of mercy?" they believe that tightening utilization controls will only increase physicians' perceived need to manipulate managed care rules in order to provide proper care.

This paper brings into the open practices that have been escalating for the past several years and are now being driven, as the authors point out, by the very nature of the reimbursement system that has evolved in the United States. An editorial that accompanies Wynia's paper, "Fidelity and Deceit at the Bedside," by Dr. Greg Bloche of the Georgetown-Johns Hopkins University Program in Law and Public Health, may be even more incisive and revealing. Dr. Bloche, who has both a medical and a law degree, notes at the outset that how doctors should act as their patient's advocate in the struggle to gain access to healthcare resources is a question not answered in the Hippocratic ethical tradition, in contemporary bioethics or in U.S. law. He reminds us that in the Hippocratic Oath, the physician pledges to prescribe regimens "for the good of my patients according to my ability and my judgment." But as any good lawyer might point out, Dr. Bloche notes, the Hippocratic Oath does not say how doctors should secure access for their patients to those prescribed regimens. The law charges physicians with duties of loyalty, including keeping confidences and avoiding conflicts of interest, but the law has not developed a duty of patient advocacy akin to a lawyer's duty of zealous advocacy in the client's behalf.

Pursuing this further, Bloche says that the scope and limits of physician advocacy with regard to healthcare payers is a new issue in the United States and is the result of hospital-based technology that, beginning back in the 1930s, put medical costs out of the reach of most Americans. But until the 1980s, insurers generally paid for whatever physicians prescribed. For the past two decades, however, healthcare plans have intervened aggressively to restrain spending and have claimed the authority and the right to reimburse only what is medically necessary. They do not, however, define in their contracts what medically necessary care is. Indeed, Bloche cites evidence that, in order to forestall lawyer-like advocacy, health plans often take the position that coverage rules are trade secrets, to be revealed neither to doctors nor to patients. Such advocacy, of course, has not been forestalled — or else we would not be discussing the Wynia or Bloche papers.

As Dr. Bloche suggests, medical necessity is open to broad interpretation and I might add that this is a prime example of the application of Werner Heisenberg's Uncertainty Principle outside the field of quantum physics. Bloche makes this very point by saying that subjectivity and scientific uncertainty in diagnosis and treatment make it impossible to write rules for every clinical circumstance. This ensures conflict over what is considered medically necessary care. Society, furthermore, has never resolved the question of whether costs should be weighed against clinical benefits, and if they should, in what manner. Such ambiguity leaves much room for health plans to be stingy in interpreting their subscribers' needs and for doctors to be vigorous in representing their patients' interest.

While conceding that the Wynia paper presents the most current reliable data on the extent to which doctors are willing to bend the rules in their patients' behalf, Dr. Bloche points to important limitations and inequities in the study. For example, he says that the term "exaggerate" (as in exaggerate the severity of the patient's condition) is pejorative in that it assumes there is a clear line of distinction between accurate and misleading clinical reporting. This belies the uncertainty and subjectivity of clinical perception and judgment. He also suggests that when the term "exaggerate" is used, it "gives short shrift to the possibility of a legitimate advocacy-oriented presentation of ambiguous clinical data." Bloche adds that gaming can vary from adroit clinical reporting to actual fabrication. The former might be within the realms of truthfulness while the latter flagrantly violates it.

Bloche asks what accounts for a doctor's willingness to deceive. He answers that a clue may lie in our profession's historical reliance on informal social norms that are inculcated during our clinical training, throughout our careers and further reinforced by interaction with professional peers. Until recently, norms imposed outside the medical community, whether by law or other sources of authority, have had little impact on the governance of medicine. While this has now changed, acceptance by the profession has been slow and incomplete. Bloche affirms that ethical fidelity to patients was the centerpiece of medical self-governance and widely regarded as desirable by society. But the transformation of the healthcare system, particularly over the past two decades, has imposed new norms and obligations that now vie with longstanding professional values and are at the root of the gaming controversy.

Bloche argues in favor of what he calls a robust conception of fidelity to patients which is rooted in the moral urgency of the people who are most vulnerable — our patients. He considers this analogous to a lawyer's commitment to his or her clients, but this does not extend to making false statements. On the other hand, a doctor's duty does include what he calls an advocacy-oriented presentation of clinical data with strategic emphasis on what is most favorable to the patient. While this duty excludes selective withholding of data, it does not obligate the doctor to follow coverage rules that are ambiguous and clearly not part of the health plan's contract. It does, however, require honoring coverage exclusions and cost-benefit tradeoff principles that are explicit in the contract. Nevertheless, I would contend that where coverage exclusions and cost-benefit tradeoffs, even within the contract, are clearly harmful to the patient or not in the patient's best interest, the doctor is obligated to make this information known to the patient and to recommend an appropriate remedy that would include bringing pressure on the insurer.

Unfortunately, no survey or editorial analysis can mitigate the enigma of what constitutes proper intensity and quality of care. There is no contract that is not open to extremes of interpretation — by the insurer to do less and by the doctor and the patient to do more. Doctors who have been inculcated since medical school are unlikely to be deterred from using every device at their disposal to provide the best possible diagnosis and treatment to each and every patient. The problems of physician manipulation of utilization and reimbursement rules on behalf of patients and the philosophic conundrum aptly posed in Bloche's editorial are unlikely to be solved until there are significant changes in the way American medicine is financed and, therefore, practiced.